Current C

Critical Care Medicine

2002-2003 Edition

Matthew Brenner, MD
Associate Professor of Medicine
Pulmonary and Critical Care Division
University of California, Irvine

Michael Safani, PharmD
Assistant Clinical Professor
School of Pharmacy
University of California, San Francisco

Georgina Heal, MD
Ryan M. Klein, MD
Scott T. Gallacher, MD
Guy Foster, MD
Michael Krutzik, MD

Farhad Mazdisnian, MD
Roham T. Zamanian, MD
Hans Poggemeyer, MD
H. L. Daneschvar, MD
S. E. Wilson, MD

Division of Pulmonary and Critical Care Medicine
College of Medicine
University of California, Irvine

Current Clinical Strategies Publishing

www.ccspublishing.com/ccs

Digital Book and Updates

Purchasers of this book may download the digital book and updates of this text at the Current Clinical Strategies Publishing Web site: www.ccspublishing.com/ccs.

Current Clinical Strategies Publishing

www.ccspublishing.com/ccs

27071 Cabot Road
Laguna Hills, California 92653
Phone: 800-331-8227
E-Mail: info@ccspublishing.com

Printed in USA

ISBN 1-929622-16-3

Contents

Advanced Cardiac Life Support

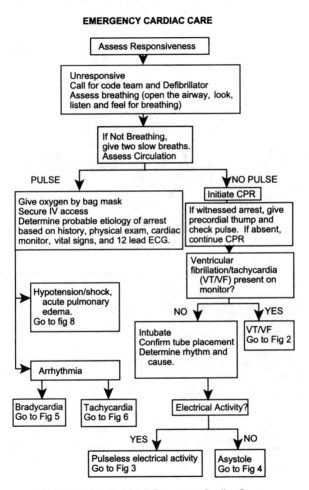

EMERGENCY CARDIAC CARE

Assess Responsiveness

Unresponsive
Call for code team and Defibrillator
Assess breathing (open the airway, look, listen and feel for breathing)

If Not Breathing,
give two slow breaths.
Assess Circulation

PULSE

NO PULSE

Give oxygen by bag mask
Secure IV access
Determine probable etiology of arrest based on history, physical exam, cardiac monitor, vital signs, and 12 lead ECG.

Initiate CPR

If witnessed arrest, give precordial thump and check pulse. If absent, continue CPR

Ventricular fibrillation/tachycardia (VT/VF) present on monitor?

NO

YES

Hypotension/shock, acute pulmonary edema.
Go to fig 8

Intubate
Confirm tube placement
Determine rhythm and cause.

VT/VF
Go to Fig 2

Arrhythmia

Bradycardia
Go to Fig 5

Tachycardia
Go to Fig 6

Electrical Activity?

YES

NO

Pulseless electrical activity
Go to Fig 3

Asystole
Go to Fig 4

Fig 1 - Algorithm for Adult Emergency Cardiac Care

**VENTRICULAR FIBRILLATION AND PULSELESS
VENTRICULAR TACHYCARDIA**

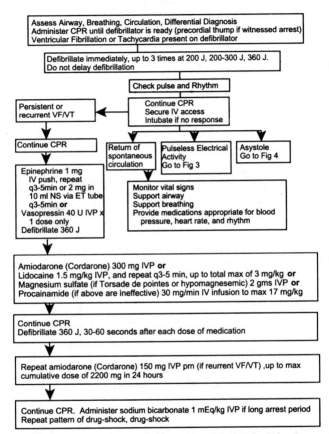

Fig 2 - Ventricular Fibrillation and Pulseless Ventricular Tachycardia

PULSELESS ELECTRICAL ACTIVITY

Pulseless Electrical Activity Includes:
    Electromechanical dissociation (EMD)
    Pseudo-EMD
    Idioventricular rhythms
    Ventricular escape rhythms
    Bradyasystolic rhythms
    Postdefibrillation idioventricular rhythms

Initiate CPR, secure IV access, intubate, assess pulse.

Determine differential diagnosis and treat underlying cause:
    Hypoxia (ventilate)
    Hypovolemia (infuse volume)
    Pericardial tamponade (performpericardiocentesis)
    Tension pneumothorax (perform needle decompression)
    Pulmonary embolism (thrombectomy, thrombolytics)
    Drug overdose with tricyclics, digoxin, beta, or calcium blockers
    Hyperkalemia or hypokalemia
    Acidosis (give bicarbonate)
    Myocardial infarction (thrombolytics)
    Hypothemia (active rewarming)

Epinephrine 1.0 mg IV bolus q3-5 min, or high dose
    epinephrine 0.1 mg/kg IV push q3-5 min; may give via
    ET tube.
Continue CPR

If bradycardia (<60 beats/min), give atroprine 1 mg IV, q3-5
    min, up to total of 0.04 mg/kg
Consider bicarbonate, 1 mEq/kg IV (1-2 amp, 44 mEq/amp),
    if hyperkalemia or other indications.

Fig 3 - Pulseless Electrical Activity

ASYSTOLE

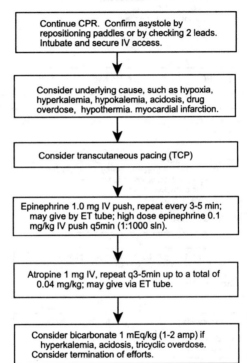

Continue CPR. Confirm asystole by repositioning paddles or by checking 2 leads. Intubate and secure IV access.

Consider underlying cause, such as hypoxia, hyperkalemia, hypokalemia, acidosis, drug overdose, hypothermia. myocardial infarction.

Consider transcutaneous pacing (TCP)

Epinephrine 1.0 mg IV push, repeat every 3-5 min; may give by ET tube; high dose epinephrine 0.1 mg/kg IV push q5min (1:1000 sln).

Atropine 1 mg IV, repeat q3-5min up to a total of 0.04 mg/kg; may give via ET tube.

Consider bicarbonate 1 mEq/kg (1-2 amp) if hyperkalemia, acidosis, tricyclic overdose. Consider termination of efforts.

Fig 4 - Asystole

BRADYCARDIA

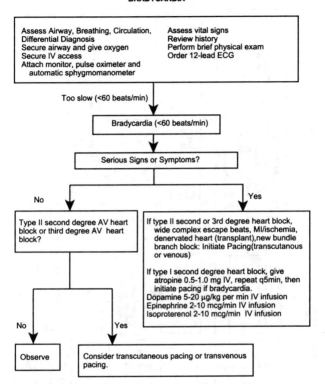

Assess Airway, Breathing, Circulation, Differential Diagnosis
Secure airway and give oxygen
Secure IV access
Attach monitor, pulse oximeter and automatic sphygmomanometer

Assess vital signs
Review history
Perform brief physical exam
Order 12-lead ECG

Too slow (<60 beats/min)

Bradycardia (<60 beats/min)

Serious Signs or Symptoms?

No

Yes

Type II second degree AV heart block or third degree AV heart block?

If type II second or 3rd degree heart block, wide complex escape beats, MI/ischemia, denervated heart (transplant),new bundle branch block: Initiate Pacing(transcutanous or venous)

If type I second degree heart block, give atropine 0.5-1.0 mg IV, repeat q5min, then initiate pacing if bradycardia.
Dopamine 5-20 µg/kg per min IV infusion
Epinephrine 2-10 mcg/min IV infusion
Isoproterenol 2-10 mcg/min IV infusion

No

Yes

Observe

Consider transcutaneous pacing or transvenous pacing.

Fig 5 - Bradycardia (with patient not in cardiac arrest).

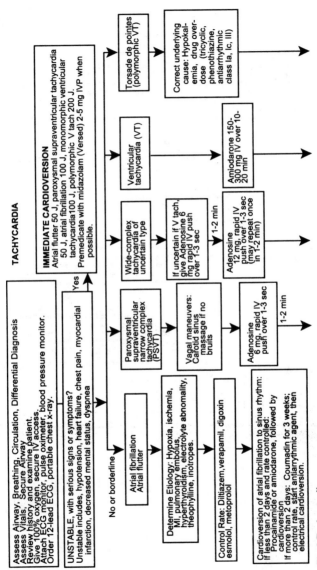

TACHYCARDIA

Assess Airway, Breathing, Circulation, Differential Diagnosis
Assess Vitals. Secure Airway
Review history, and examine patient.
Give 100% oxygen, secure IV access.
Attach ECG monitor, pulse oximeter, blood pressure monitor.
Order 12-lead ECG, portable chest x-ray.

UNSTABLE, with serious signs or symptoms?
Unstable includes, hypotension, heart failure, chest pain, myocardial infarction, decreased mental status, dyspnea

No or borderline

Yes →

IMMEDIATE CARDIOVERSION
Atrial flutter 50 J, paroxysmal supraventricular tachycardia 50 J, atrial fibrillation 100 J, monomorphic ventricular tachycardia100 J, polymorphic V tach 200 J. Premedicate with midazolam (Versed) 2-5 mg IVP when possible.

↓

Atrial fibrillation / Atrial flutter

Determine Etiology: Hypoxia, ischemia, MI, pulmonary embolus, hyperthyroidism, electrolyte abnormality, theophylline, inotropes.

Control Rate: Diltiazem, verapamil, digoxin esmolol, metoprolol

Cardioversion of atrial fibrillation to sinus rhythm: If less than 2 days and rate controlled: Procainamide or amiodarone, followed by cardioversion
If more than 2 days: Coumadin for 3 weeks; control rate, start antiarrhythmic agent, then electrical cardioversion.

Paroxysmal supraventricular narrow complex tachycardia (PSVT)

Vagal maneuvers: Carotid sinus massage if no bruits

Adenosine 6 mg, rapid IV push over 1-3 sec

1-2 min
→

Wide-complex tachycardia of uncertain type

If uncertain if V tach, give Adenosine 6 mg rapid IV push over 1-3 sec

1-2 min

Adenosine 12 mg, rapid IV push over 1-3 sec (may repeat once in 1-2 min)
→

Ventricular tachycardia (VT)

Amiodarone 150-300 mg IV over 10-20 min
→

Torsade de pointes (polymorphic VT)

Correct underlying cause: Hypokalemia, drug overdose (tricyclic, phenothiazine, antiarrhythmic class Ia, Ic, III)
→

Fig 6 Tachycardia

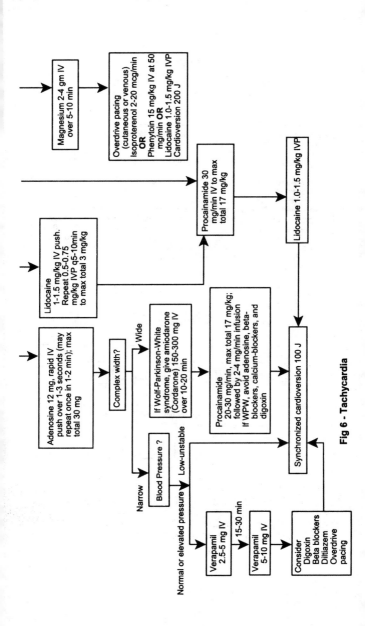

Magnesium 2-4 gm IV over 5-10 min

Overdrive pacing (cutaneous or venous) Isoproterenol 2-20 mcg/min **OR** Phenytoin 15 mg/kg IV at 50 mg/min **OR** Lidocaine 1.0-1.5 mg/kg IVP Cardioversion 200 J

Procainamide 30 mg/min IV to max total 17 mg/kg

Lidocaine 1.0-1.5 mg/kg IVP

Lidocaine 1-1.5 mg/kg IV push. Repeat once in 1-2 min); max total 30 mg/kg IVP q5-10min to max total 3 mg/kg

Adenosine 12 mg, rapid IV push over 1-3 seconds (may repeat once in 1-2 min); max total 30 mg

Complex width?

Wide

Narrow

If Wolf-Parkinson-White syndrome, give amiodarone (Cordarone) 150-300 mg IV over 10-20 min

Procainamide 20-30 mg/min, max total 17 mg/kg; followed by 2-4 mg/min infusion If WPW, avoid adenosine, beta-blockers, calcium-blockers, and digoxin

Blood Pressure ?

Low-unstable

Normal or elevated pressure

Synchronized cardioversion 100 J

Verapamil 2.5-5 mg IV

15-30 min

Verapamil 5-10 mg IV

Consider Digoxin Beta blockers Diltiazem Overdrive pacing

Fig 6 - Tachycardia

STABLE TACHYCARDIA

Stable tachycardia with serious signs and symptoms related to the tachycardia. Patient not in cardiac arrest.

↓

If ventricular rate is >150 beats/min, prepare for immediate cardioversion.
Treatment of Stable Patients is based on Arrhythmia Type:

Ventricular Tachycardia:
Procainamide (Pronestyl) 30 mg/min IV, up to a total max of 17 mg/kg, or
Amiodarone (Cordarone) 150-300 mg IV over 10-20 min, or
Lidocaine 0.75 mg/kg. Procainamide should be avoided if ejection fraction is <40%.

Paroxysmal Supraventricular Tachycardia: Carotid sinus pressure (if bruits absent), then adenosine 6 mg rapid IVP, followed by 12 mg rapid IVP x 2 doses to max total 30 mg. If no response, verapamil 2.5-5.0 mg IVP; may repeat dose with 5-10 mg IVP if adequate blood pressure; or Esmolol 500 mcg/kg IV over 1 min, then 50 mcg/kg/min IV infusion, and titrate up to 200 mcg/kg/min IV infusion.

Atrial Fibrillation/Flutter:
Ejection fraction ≥40%: Diltiazem (Cardizem) 0.25 mg/kg IV over 2 min; may repeat 0.35 mg/kg IV over 2 min prn x 1 to control rate. Then give procainamide (Pronestyl) 30 mg/min IV infusion, up to a total max of 17 mg/kg
Ejection fraction <40%: Digoxin 0.5 mg IVP, then 0.25 mg IVP q4h x 2 to control rate. Then give amiodarone (Cordarone) 150-300 mg IV over 10-20 min.

↓

Check oxygen saturation, suction device, intubation equipment. Secure IV access

↓

Premedicate whenever possible with Midazolam (Versed) 2-5 mg IVP or sodium pentothal 2 mg/kg rapid IVP

↓

Synchronized cardioversion

Atrialflutter	50 J
PSVT	50 J
Atrial	100 J
Monomorphic V-tach	100 J
Polymorphic V tach	200 J

Fig 7 - Stable Tachycardia (not in cardiac arrest)

HYPOTENSION, SHOCK, AND ACUTE PULMONARY EDEMA

Signs and symptoms of congestive heart failure, acute pulmonary edema.
Assess ABCD's, secure airway, administer oxygen; secure IV access. Monitor ECG, pulse oximeter,
blood pressure, order 12-lead ECG, portable chest X-ray,
Check vital signs, review history, and examine patient. Determine differential diagnosis.

Determine underlying cause

Hypovolemia

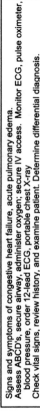

Administer Fluids, Blood
Consider vasopressors
Apply hemostasis; treat
underlying problem

Pump Failure

Determine blood pressure

Systolic BP
<70 mm Hg

Norepinephrine 0.5-
30 µg/min IV or
Dopamine 5-20 µg/kg
per min

Systolic BP
70-100 mm Hg

Dopamine 2.5-20
µg/kg per min IV
(add norepinephrine
if dopamine is >20
µg/kg per min)

Systolic BP >100 mm Hg
and diastolic BP normal

Dobutamine 2.0-20
µg/kg per min IV

Furosemide IV 0.5-1.0 mg/kg
Morphine IV 1-3 mg
Nitroglycerin SL 0.4 mg tab
q3-5min x3
Oxygen

Bradycardia or Tachycardia

Bradycardia
Go to Fig 5

Tachycardia
Go to Fig 6

Diastolic BP >110 mm Hg

If ischemia and hypertension:
Nitroglycerin10-20 µg/min
IV, and titrate to effect and/or
Nitroprusside 0.1-5.0
µg/kg/min IV

Fig 8 - Hypotension, Shock, and Acute Pulmonary Edema

Critical Care Patient Management

T. Scott Gallacher, MD, MS

Critical Care History and Physical Examination

Chief complaint: Reason for admission to the ICU.

History of present illness: This section should included pertinent chronological events leading up to the hospitalization. It should include events during hospitalization and eventual admission to the ICU.

Prior cardiac history: Angina (stable, unstable, changes in frequency), exacerbating factors (exertional, rest angina). History of myocardial infarction, heart failure, coronary artery bypass graft surgery, angioplasty. Previous exercise treadmill testing, ECHO, ejection fraction. Request old ECG, ECHO, impedance cardiography, stress test results, and angiographic studies.

Chest pain characteristics:

A. **Pain:** Quality of pain, pressure, squeezing, tightness

B. **Onset of pain:** Exertional, awakening from sleep, relationship to activities of daily living (ADLs), such as eating, walking, bathing, and grooming.

C. **Severity and quality:** Pressure, tightness, sharp, pleuritic

D. **Radiation:** Arm, jaw, shoulder

E. **Associated symptoms:** Diaphoresis, dyspnea, back pain, GI symptoms.

F. **Duration:** Minutes, hours, days.

G. **Relieving factors:** Nitroclycerine, rest.

Cardiac risk factors: Age, male, diabetes, hypercholesteremia, low HDL, hypertension, smoking, previous coronary artery disease, family history of arteriosclerosis (eg, myocardial infarction in males less than 50 years old, stroke).

Congestive heart failure symptoms: Orthopnea (number of pillows), paroxysmal nocturnal dyspnea, dyspnea on exertional, edema.

Peripheral vascular disease symptoms: Claudication, transient ischemic attack, cerebral vascular accident.

COPD exacerbation symptoms: Shortness of breath, fever, chills, wheezing, sputum production, hemoptysis (quantify), corticosteroid use, previous intubation.

Past medical history: Peptic ulcer disease, renal disease, diabetes, COPD. Functional status prior to hospitalization.

Medications: Dose and frequency. Use of nitroglycerine, beta-agonist, steroids.

Allergies: Penicillin, contrast dye, aspirin; describe the specific reaction (eg, anaphylaxis, wheezing, rash, hypotension).

Social history: Tobacco use, alcohol consumption, intravenous drug use.

Review of systems: Review symptoms related to each organ system.

Critical Care Physical Examination

Vital signs:

Temperature, pulse, respiratory rate, BP (vital signs should be given in ranges)

Input/Output: IV fluid volume/urine output.

Special parameters: Oxygen saturation, pulmonary artery wedge pressure (PAWP), systemic vascular resistance (SVR), ventilator settings, impedance cardiography.

General: Mental status, Glasgow coma score, degree of distress.

HEENT: PERRLA, EOMI, carotid pulse.

Lungs: Inspection, percussion, auscultation for wheezes, crackles.

Cardiac: Lateral displacement of point of maximal impulse; irregular rate,, irregular rhythm (atrial fibrillation); S3 gallop (LV dilation), S4 (myocardial infarction), holosystolic apex murmur (mitral regurgitation).

Cardiac murmurs: 1/6 = faint; 2/6 = clear; 3/6 - loud; 4/6 = palpable; 5/6 = heard with stethoscope off the chest; 6/6 = heard without stethoscope.

Abdomen: Bowel sounds normoactive, abdomen soft and nontender.

Extremities: Cyanosis, clubbing, edema, peripheral pulses 2+.

Skin: Capillary refill, skin turgor.

Neuro

Deficits in strength, sensation.

Deep tendon reflexes: 0 = absent; 1 = diminished; 2 = normal; 3 = brisk; 4 = hyperactive clonus.

Motor Strength: 0 = no contractility; 1 = contractility but no joint motion; 2 = motion without gravity; 3 = motion against gravity; 4 = motion against some resistance; 5 = motion against full resistance (normal).

Labs: CBC, INR/PTT; chem 7, chem 12, Mg, $pH/pCO_2/pO_2$. CXR, ECG, impedance cardiography, other diagnostic studies.

Impression/Problem list: Discuss diagnosis and plan for each problem by system.

Neurologic Problems: List and discuss neurologic problems

Pulmonary Problems: Ventilator management.

Cardiac Problems: Arrhythmia, chest pain, angina.

GI Problems: H2 blockers, nasogastric tubes, nutrition.

Genitourinary and Electrolytes Problems: Fluid status: IV fluids, electrolyte therapy.

Hematologic Problems: Blood or blood products, DVT prophylaxis.

Infectious Disease: Plans for antibiotic therapy; antibiotic day number, culture results.

Endocrine/Nutrition: Serum glucose control, parenteral or enteral nutrition, diet.

Admission Check List

1. **Call and request** old chart, ECG, and x-rays.
2. **Stat labs:** CBC, chem 7, cardiac enzymes (myoglobin, troponin, CPK), INR, PTT, C&S, ABG, UA, cardiac enzymes (myoglobin, troponin, CPK).
3. **Labs:** Toxicology screens and drug levels.
4. **Cultures:** Blood culture x 2, urine and sputum culture (before initiating antibiotics), sputum Gram stain, urinalysis.
5. **CXR, ECG**, diagnostic studies.
6. **Discuss case with resident, attending**, and family.

Critical Care Progress Note

ICU Day Number:
Antibiotic Day Number:
Subjective: Patient is awake and alert. Note any events that occurred overnight.
Objective: Temperature, maximum temperature, pulse, respiratory rate, BP, 24-hr input and output, pulmonary artery pressure, pulmonary capillary wedge pressure, cardiac output.
Lungs: Clear bilaterally
Cardiac: Regular rate and rhythm, no murmur, no rubs.
Abdomen: Bowel sounds normoactive, soft-nontender.
Neuro: No local deficits in strength, sensation.
Extremities: No cyanosis, clubbing, edema, peripheral pulses 2+.
Labs: CBC, ABG, chem 7.
ECG: **Chest x-ray:**
Impression and Plan: Give an overall impression, and then discuss impression and plan by organ system:
    Cardiovascular:
    Pulmonary:
    Neurological:
    Gastrointestinal:
    Infectious:
    Endocrine:
    Nutrition:

Procedure Note

A procedure note should be written in the chart when a procedure is performed. Procedure notes are brief operative notes.

Procedure Note

Date and time:
Procedure:
Indications:
Patient Consent: Document that the indications, risks and alternatives to the procedure were explained to the patient. Note that the patient was given the opportunity to ask questions and that the patient consented to the procedure in writing.
Lab tests: Relevant labs, such as the INR and CBC
Anesthesia: Local with 2% lidocaine
Description of Procedure: Briefly describe the procedure, including sterile prep, anesthesia method, patient position, devices used, anatomic location of procedure, and outcome.
Complications and Estimated Blood Loss (EBL):
Disposition: Describe how the patient tolerated the procedure.
Specimens: Describe any specimens obtained and labs tests which were ordered.
Name of Physician: Name of person performing procedure and supervising staff.

Discharge Note

The discharge note should be written in the patient's chart prior to discharge.

Discharge Note
Date/time: **Diagnoses:** **Treatment:** Briefly describe therapy provided during hospitalization, including surgical procedures and antibiotic therapy. **Studies Performed:** Electrocardiograms, CT scans. **Discharge medications:** **Follow-up Arrangements:**

Fluids and Electrolytes

Maintenance Fluids Guidelines:
    70 kg Adult: D5 1/4 NS with 20 mEq KCl/Liter at 125 mL/hr.
Specific Replacement Fluids for Specific Losses:
    Gastric (nasogastric tube, emesis): D5 ½ NS with 20 mEq/L KCL.
    Diarrhea: D5LR with 15 mEq/liter KCl. Provide 1 liter of replacement for each 1 kg or 2.2 lb of body weight lost.
    Bile: D5LR with 25 mEq/liter (½ amp) of sodium bicarbonate.
    Pancreatic: D5LR with 50 mEq/liter (1 amp) sodium bicarbonate.

Blood Component Therapy

A. **Packed red blood cells (PRBCs).** Each unit provides 250-400 cc of volume, and each unit should raise hemoglobin by 1 gm/dL and hematocrit by 3%. PRBCs are usually requested in two unit increments.

B. **Type and screen.** Blood is tested for A, B, Rh antigens, and antibodies to donor erythrocytes. If blood products are required, the blood can be rapidly prepared by the blood bank. O negative blood is used when type and screen information is not available, but the need for transfusion is emergent.

C. **Type and cross match** sets aside specific units of packed donor red blood cells. If blood is needed on an urgent basis, type and cross should be requested.

D. **Platelets.** Indicated for bleeding if there is thrombocytopenia or platelet dysfunction in the setting of uncontrolled bleeding. Each unit of platelet concentrate should raise the platelet count by 5,000-10,000. Platelets are usually transfused 6-10 units at a time, which should increase the platelet count by 40-60,000. Thrombocytopenia is defined as a platelet count of less than 60,000. For surgery, the count should be greater than 50,000.

E. **Fresh Frozen Plasma (FFP)** is used for active bleeding secondary to liver disease, warfarin overdose, dilutional coagulopathy secondary to multiple blood transfusions, disseminated intravascular coagulopathy, and vitamin K and coagulation factor deficiencies. Administration of FFP requires ABO typing, but not cross matching.

1. Each unit contains coagulation factors in normal concentration.
2. Two to four units are usually required for therapeutic intervention.

F. **Cryoprecipitate**
   1. Indicated in patients with Hemophilia A, Von Willebrand's disease, and any state of hypofibrinogenemia requiring replacement (DIC), or reversal of thrombolytic therapy.
   2. Cryoprecipitate contains factor VIII, fibrinogen, and Von Willebrand factor. The goal of therapy is to maintain the fibrinogen level above 100 mL/dL, which is usually achieved with 10 units given over 3-5 minutes.

Total Parenteral Nutrition

Infuse 40-50 mL/hr of amino acid dextrose solution in the first 24 hr; increase daily by 40 mL/hr increments until providing 1.3-2 x basal energy requirement and 1.2-1.7 gm protein/kg/d (see formula, page 145)

Standard Solution per Liter

Amino acid solution (Aminosyn) 7-10%	500 mL
Dextrose 40-70%	500 mL
Sodium	35 mEq
Potassium	36 mEq
Chloride	35 mEq
Calcium	4.5 mEq
Phosphate	9 mMol
Magnesium	8.0 mEq
Acetate	82-104 mEq
Multi-Trace Element Formula	1 mL/d
Regular insulin (if indicated)	10-20 U/L
Multivitamin 12 (2 amp)	10 mL/d
Vitamin K (in solution, SQ, IM)	10 mg/week
Vitamin B 12	1000 mcg/week

Fat Emulsion:
-Intralipid 20% 500 mL/d IVPB infused in parallel with standard solution at 1 mL/min x 15 min; if no adverse reactions, increase to 20-50 mL/hr. Serum triglyceride level should be checked 6h after end of infusion (maintain <250 mg/dL).

Cyclic Total Parenteral Nutrition
-12-hour night schedule; taper continuous infusion in morning by reducing rate to half original rate for 1 hour. Further reduce rate by half for an additional hour, then discontinue. Restart TPN in evening. Taper at beginning and end of cycle. Final rate should be 185 mL/hr for 9-10h with 2 hours of taper at each end, for total of 2000 mL.

Peripheral Parenteral Supplementation
-Amino acid solution (ProCalamine) 3% up to 3 L/d at 125 cc/h OR
-Combine 500 mL amino acid solution 7% or 10% (Aminosyn) and 500 mL 20% dextrose and electrolyte additive. Infuse at up to 100 cc/hr in parallel with intralipid 10% or 20% at 1 mL/min for 15 min (test dose); if no adverse reactions, infuse 500 mL/d at 20 mL/hr.

Special Medications
-Famotidine (Pepcid) 20 mg IV q12h or 40 mg/day in TPN **OR**
-Ranitidine (Zantac) 50 mg IV q6-8h.
-Insulin sliding scale or continuous IV infusion.

Labs
Baseline: Draw labs below. Chest x-ray, plain film for tube placement
Daily Labs: Chem 7, osmolality, CBC, cholesterol, triglyceride (6h after end of infusion), serum phosphate, magnesium, calcium, urine specific gravity.
Weekly Labs: Protein, iron, TIBC, INR/PTT, 24h urine nitrogen and creatinine. Pre-albumin, transferrin, albumin, total protein, AST, ALT, GGT, alkaline phosphatase, LDH, amylase, total bilirubin.

Enteral Nutrition

General Measures: Daily weights, nasoduodenal feeding tube. Head of bed at 30 degrees while enteral feeding and 2 hours after completion. Record bowel movements.

Continuous Enteral Infusion: Initial enteral solution (Osmolite, Pulmocare, Jevity) 30 mL/hr. Measure residual volume q1h x 12h, then tid; hold feeding for 1 h if residual is more than 100 mL of residual. Increase rate by 25-50 mL/hr at 24 hr intervals as tolerated until final rate of 50-100 mL/hr (1 cal/mL) as tolerated. Three tablespoons of protein powder (Promix) may be added to each 500 cc of solution. Flush tube with 100 cc water q8h.

Enteral Bolus Feeding: Give 50-100 mL of enteral solution (Osmolite, Pulmocare, Jevity) q3h initially. Increase amount in 50 mL steps to max of 250-300 mL q3-4h; 30 kcal of nonprotein calories/d and 1.5 gm protein/kg/d. Before each feeding measure residual volume, and delay feeding by 1 h if >100 mL. Flush tube with 100 cc of water after each bolus.

Special Medications:
-Metoclopramide (Reglan) 10-20 mg PO, IM, IV, or in J tube q6h.
-Famotidine (Pepcid) 20 mg J-tube q12h **OR**
-Ranitidine (Zantac) 150 mg in J-tube bid.

Symptomatic Medications:
-Loperamide (Imodium) 24 mg PO or in J-tube q6h, max 16 mg/d prn **OR**
-Diphenoxylate/atropine (Lomotil) 5-10 mL (2.5 mg/5 mL) PO or in J-tube q4-6h, max 12 tabs/d **OR**
-Kaopectate 30 cc PO or in J-tube q6h.

Radiographic Evaluation of Interventions

I. **Central intravenous lines**
    A. **Central venous catheters** should be located well above the right atrium, and not in a neck vein. Rule out pneumothorax by checking that the lung markings extend completely to the rib cages on both sides. Examine for hydropericardium ("water bottle" sign, mediastinal widening).
    B. **Pulmonary artery catheter tips** should be located centrally and posteriorly, and not more than 3-5 cm from midline.
II. **Endotracheal tubes.** Verify that the tube is located 3 cm below the vocal cords and 2-4cm above the carina; the tip of tube should be at the level of aortic arch.

III. **Tracheostomies.** Verify by chest x-ray that the tube is located halfway between the stoma and the carina; the tube should be parallel to the long axis of the trachea. The tube should be approximately 2/3 of width of the trachea; the cuff should not cause bulging of the trachea walls. Check for subcutaneous air in the neck tissue and for mediastinal widening secondary to air leakage.

IV. **Nasogastric tubes and feeding tubes.** Verify that the tube is in the stomach and not coiled in the esophagus or trachea. The tip of the tube should not be near the gastroesophageal junction.

V. **Chest tubes.** A chest tube for pneumothorax drainage should be near the level of the third intercostal space. If the tube is intended to drain a free-flowing pleural effusion, it should be located inferior-posteriorly, at or about the level of the eighth intercostal space. Verify that the side port of the tube is within the thorax.

VI. **Mechanical ventilation.** Obtain a chest x-ray to rule out pneumothorax, subcutaneous emphysema, pneumomediastinum, or subpleural air cysts. Lung infiltrates or atelectasis may diminish or disappear after initiation of mechanical ventilation because of increased aeration of the affected lung lobe.

Arterial Line Placement

Procedure

1. Obtain a 20-gauge 1 ½-2 inch catheter over needle assembly (Angiocath), arterial line setup (transducer, tubing and pressure bag containing heparinized saline), arm board, sterile dressing, lidocaine, 3 cc syringe, 25-gauge needle, and 3-O silk suture.

2. The radial artery is the most frequently used artery. Use the Allen test to verify the patency of the radial and ulnar arteries. Place the extremity on an arm board with a gauze roll behind the wrist to maintain hyperextension.

3. Prep the skin with povidone-iodine and drape; infiltrate 1% lidocaine using a 25-gauge needle. Choose a site where the artery is most superficial and distal.

4. Palpate the artery with the left hand, and advance the catheter-over-needle assembly into the artery at a 30-degree angle to the skin. When a flash of blood is seen, hold the needle in place and advance the catheter into the artery. Occlude the artery with manual pressure while the pressure tubing is connected.

5. Advance the guide wire into the artery, and pass the catheter over the guide wire. Suture the catheter in place with 3-0 silk and apply dressing.

Central Venous Catheterization

I. **Indications for central venous catheter cannulation:** Monitoring of central venous pressures in shock or heart failure; management of fluid status; insertion of a transvenous pacemaker; administration of total parenteral nutrition; administration of vesicants (chemotherapeutic agents).

II. **Location:** The internal jugular approach is relatively contraindicated in patients with a carotid bruit, stenosis, or an aneurysm. The subclavian approach has an increased risk of pneumothorax in patients with emphysema or bullae. The external jugular or internal jugular approach is preferable in patients with coagulopathy or thrombocytopenia because of the ease of external compression. In patients with unilateral lung pathology or a chest tube already in place, the catheter should be placed on the side of predominant pathology or on the side with the chest tube if present.

III. Technique for insertion of external jugular vein catheter

1. The external jugular vein extends from the angle of the mandible to behind the middle of the clavicle, where it joins with the subclavian vein. Place the patient in Trendelenburg's position. Cleanse skin with Betadine-iodine solution, and, using sterile technique, inject 1% lidocaine to produce a skin weal. Apply digital pressure to the external jugular vein above the clavicle to distend the vein.

2. With a 16-gauge thin wall needle, advance the needle into the vein. Then pass a J-guide wire through the needle; the wire should advance without resistance. Remove the needle, maintaining control over the guide wire at all times. Nick the skin with a No. 11 scalpel blade.

3. With the guide wire in place, pass the central catheter over the wire and remove the guide wire after the catheter is in place. Cover the catheter hub with a finger to prevent air embolization.

4. Attach a syringe to the catheter hub and ensure that there is free back-flow of dark venous blood. Attach the catheter to an intravenous infusion.

5. Secure the catheter in place with 2-0 silk suture and tape. The catheter should be replaced weekly or if there is any sign of infection.

6. Obtain a chest x-ray to confirm position and rule out pneumothorax.

IV. Internal jugular vein cannulation.
The internal jugular vein is positioned behind the sternocleidomastoid muscle lateral to the carotid artery. The catheter should be placed at a location at the upper confluence of the two bellies of the sternocleidomastoid, at the level of the cricoid cartilage.

1. Place the patient in Trendelenburg's position and turn the patient's head to the contralateral side.

2. Choose a location on the right or left. If lung function is symmetrical and no chest tubes are in place, the right side is preferred because of the direct path to the superior vena cava. Prepare the skin with Betadine solution using sterile technique and placea drape. Infiltrate the skin and deeper tissues with 1% lidocaine.

3. Palpate the carotid artery. Using a 22-gauge scout needle and syringe, direct the needle lateral to the carotid artery towards the ipsilateral nipple at a 30-degree angle to the neck. While aspirating, advance the needle until the vein is located and blood flows back into the syringe.

4. Remove the scout needle and advance a 16-gauge, thin wall catheter-over-needle with an attached syringe along the same path as the scout needle. When back flow of blood is noted into the syringe, advance the catheter into the vein. Remove the needle and confirm back flow of blood through the catheter and into the syringe. Remove the syringe, and use a finger to cover the catheter hub to prevent air embolization.

5. With the 16-gauge catheter in position, advance a 0.89 mm x 45 cm spring guide wire through the catheter. The guidewire should advance easily without resistance.

6. With the guidewire in position, remove the catheter and use a No. 11 scalpel blade to nick the skin.

7. Place the central vein catheter over the wire, holding the wire secure at all times. Pass the catheter into the vein, remove the guidewire, and suture the catheter with 0 silk suture, tape, and connect it to an IV infusion.

8. Obtain a chest x-ray to rule out pneumothorax and confirm position of the catheter.

V. Subclavian vein cannulation. The subclavian vein is located in the angle formed by the medial 1/3 of the clavicle and the first rib.

1. Position the patient supine with a rolled towel located between the patient's scapulae, and turn the patient's head towards the contralateral side. Prepare the area with Betadine iodine solution, and, using sterile technique, drape the area and infiltrate 1% lidocaine into the skin and tissues.

2. Advance the 16-gauge catheter-over-needle, with syringe attached, into a location inferior to the mid-point of the clavicle, until the clavicle bone and needle come in contact.

3. Slowly probe down with the needle until the needle slips under the clavicle, and advance it slowly towards the vein until the catheter needle enters the vein and a back flow of venous blood enters the syringe. Remove the syringe, and cover the catheter hub with a finger to prevent air embolization.

4. With the 16-gauge catheter in position, advance a 0.89 mm x 45 cm spring guide wire through the catheter. The guide wire should advance easily without resistance.

5. With the guide wire in position, remove the catheter, and use a No. 11 scalpel blade to nick the skin.

6. Place the central line catheter over the wire, holding the wire secure at all times. Pass the catheter into the vein, and suture the catheter with 2-0 silk suture, tape, and connect to an IV infusion.

7. Obtain a chest x-ray to confirm position and rule out pneumothorax.

VI. Pulmonary artery catheterization

1. Using sterile technique, cannulate a vein using the technique above. The subclavian vein or internal jugular vein is commonly used.

2. Advance a guide wire through the cannula, then remove the cannula, but leave the guide wire in place. Keep the guide wire under control at all times. Nick the skin with a number 11 scalpel blade adjacent to the guide wire, and pass a number 8 French introducer over the wire into the vein. Remove the wire and connect the introducer to an IV fluid infusion, and suture with 2-0 silk.

3. Pass the proximal end of the pulmonary artery catheter (Swan Ganz) to an assistant for connection to a continuous flush transducer system.

4. Flush the distal and proximal ports with heparin solution, remove all bubbles, and check balloon integrity by inflating 2 cc of air. Check the pressure transducer by quickly moving the distal tip and watching the monitor for response.

5. Pass the catheter through the introducer into the vein, then inflate the balloon with 1.0 cc of air, and advance the catheter until the balloon is in or near the right atrium.

6. The approximate distance to the entrance of the right atrium is determined from the site of insertion:
   Right internal jugular vein: 10-15 cm.
   Subclavian vein: 10 cm.
   Femoral vein: 35.45 cm.

7. Advance the inflated balloon, while monitoring pressures and wave forms as the PA catheter is advanced. Advance the catheter through the right ventricle into the main pulmonary artery until the catheter enters a distal

branch of the pulmonary artery and is stopped (as evidenced by a pulmonary wedge pressure waveform).

8. Do not advance the catheter while the balloon is deflated, and do not withdraw the catheter with the balloon inflated. After placement, obtain a chest X-ray to ensure that the tip of catheter is no farther than 3-5 cm from the mid-line, and no pneumothorax is present.

Normal Pulmonary Artery Catheter Values

Right atrial pressure	1-7 mm Hg
RVP systolic	15-25 mm Hg
RVP diastolic	8-15 mm Hg
Pulmonary artery pressure	
PAP systolic	15-25 mm Hg
PAP diastolic	8-15 mm Hg
PAP mean	10-20 mm Hg

Cardiovascular Disorders

Roham T. Zamanian, MD
Farhad Mazdisnian, MD
Michael Krutzik, MD

Acute Coronary Syndromes (Acute Myocardial Infarction and Unstable Angina)

Acute myocardial infarction (AMI) and unstable angina are part of a spectrum known as the acute coronary syndromes (ACS), which have in common a ruptured atheromatous plaque. These syndromes include unstable angina, non–Q-wave MI, and Q-wave MI. The ECG presentation of ACS includes ST-segment elevation infarction, ST-segment depression (including non–Q-wave MI and unstable angina), and nondiagnostic ST-segment and T-wave abnormalities. Patients with ST-segment elevation will usually develop Q-wave MI. Patients with ischemic chest discomfort who do not have ST-segment elevation will develop Q-wave MI and non–Q-wave MI or unstable angina.

I. **Clinical evaluation of chest pain and acute coronary syndromes**
    A. **History.** Chest pain is present in 69% of patients with AMI. The pain may be characterized as a constricting or squeezing sensation in the chest. Pain can radiate to the upper abdomen, back, either arm, either shoulder, neck, or jaw. Atypical pain presentations in AMI include pleuritic, sharp or burning chest pain. Dyspnea, nausea, vomiting, palpitations, or syncope may be the only complaints.
    B. **Cardiac Risk factors** include hypertension, hyperlipidemia, diabetes, smoking, and a strong family history (coronary artery disease in early or mid-adulthood in a first-degree relative).
    C. **Physical examination** may reveal tachycardia or bradycardia, hyper- or hypotension, or tachypnea. Inspiratory rales and an S3 gallop are associated with left-sided failure. Jugulovenous distention (JVD), hepatojugular reflux, and peripheral edema suggest right-sided failure. A systolic murmur may indicate ischemic mitral regurgitation or ventricular septal defect.

II. **Laboratory evaluation of chest pain and acute coronary syndromes**
    A. **Electrocardiogram (ECG).** The initial ECG reveals diagnostic ST elevations in only 40% of patients with a confirmed AMI. ST-segment elevation (equal to or greater than 1 mV) in two or more contiguous leads provides strong evidence of thrombotic coronary arterial occlusion and makes the patient a candidate for immediate reperfusion by thrombolysis or angioplasty.
    B. **Laboratory markers**
        1. **Creatine phosphokinase** (CPK) enzyme is found in the brain, muscle, and heart. The cardiac-specific dimer, CK-MB, however, is present almost exclusively in myocardium.

Common Markers for Acute Myocardial Infarction			
Marker	Initial Elevation After MI	Mean Time to Peak Elevations	Time to Return to Baseline
Myoglobin	1-4 h	6-7 h	18-24 h
CTnI	3-12 h	10-24 h	3-10 d
CTnT	3-12 h	12-48 h	5-14 d
CKMB	4-12 h	10-24 h	48-72 h
CKMBiso	2-6 h	12 h	38 h

CTnI, CTnT = troponins of cardiac myofibrils; CPK-MB, MM = tissue isoforms of creatine kinase.

2. **CK-MB subunits.** Subunits of CK, CK-MB, -MM, and -BB, are markers associated with a release into the blood from damaged cells. Elevated CK-MB enzyme levels are observed in the serum 2-6 hours after MI, but may not be detected until up to 12 hours after the onset of symptoms.

3. **Cardiac-specific troponin T (cTnT)** is a qualitative assay and cardiac troponin I (cTnI) is a quantitative assay. The cTnT level remains elevated in serum up to 14 days and cTnI for 3-7 days after infarction.

4. **Myoglobin** is the first cardiac enzyme to be released. It appears earlier but is less specific for MI than other markers. Myoglobin is most useful for ruling out myocardial infarction in the first few hours.

III. Initial treatment of acute coronary syndromes

A. **Continuous cardiac monitoring and IV access** should be initiated. **Morphine, oxygen, nitroglycerin, and aspirin ("MONA")** should be administered to patients with ischemic-type chest pain unless contraindicated.

B. **Morphine** is indicated for continuing pain unresponsive to nitrates. Morphine reduces ventricular preload and oxygen requirements by venodilation. Administer morphine sulfate 2-4 mg IV every 5-10 minutes prn for pain or anxiety.

C. **Oxygen** should be administered to all patients with ischemic-type chest discomfort and suspected ACS for at least 2 to 3 hours.

D. **Nitroglycerin**
1. Nitroglycerin is an analgesic for ischemic-type chest discomfort. Nitroglycerin is indicated for the initial management of pain and ischemia unless contraindicated by hypotension (SBP <90 mm Hg) or RV infarction. Continued use of nitroglycerin beyond 48 hours is only indicated for recurrent angina or pulmonary congestion.
2. Initially, give up to three doses of 0.4 mg sublingual NTG every five minutes or nitroglycerine aerosol, 1 spray sublingually every 5 minutes. An infusion of intravenous NTG may be started at 10-20

mcg/min, titrating upward by 5-10 mcg/min every 5-10 minutes (maximum, 3 mcg/kg/min). Titrate to decrease the mean arterial pressure by 10% in normotensive patients and by 30% in those with hypertension. Slow or stop the infusion if the SBP drops below 100 mm Hg.

E. **Aspirin**
   1. Aspirin should be given as soon as possible to all patients with suspected ACS unless the patient is allergic to it. Aspirin therapy reduces mortality after MI by 25%.
   2. A dose of 160-325 mg of aspirin should be chewed and swallowed on day 1 and continued PO daily thereafter. If aspirin is contraindicated, clopidogrel (Plavix) 75 mg qd should be administered.

IV. **Risk stratification, initial therapy, and evaluation for reperfusion in the emergency department**

Risk Stratification with the First 12-Lead ECG

Use the 12-lead ECG to triage patients into 1 of 3 groups:
   1. ST-segment elevation
   2. ST-segment depression(≥1 mm)
   3. Nondiagnostic or normal ECG

A. Patients with ischemic-type chest pain and ST-segment elevation ≥1 mm in 2 contiguous leads have acute myocardial infarction. Reperfusion therapy with thrombolytics or angioplasty is recommended.

B. Patients with ischemic-type pain but normal or nondiagnostic ECGs or ECGs consistent with ischemia (ST-segment depression only) usually do not have AMI. These patients should not be given fibrinolytic therapy.

C. Patients with normal or nondiagnostic ECGs usually do not have AMI, and they should be evaluated with serial cardiac enzymes and additional tests to determine the cause of their symptoms.

V. **Management of ST-segment elevation myocardial infarction**

A. Patients with ST-segment elevation have AMI should receive reperfusion therapy with fibrinolytics or percutaneous coronary intervention.

B. **Reperfusion therapy: Fibrinolytics**
   1. Patients who present with ischemic pain and ST-segment elevation (≥1 mm in ≥2 contiguous leads) within 12 hours of onset of persistent pain should receive fibrinolytic therapy unless contraindicated. Patients with a new bundle branch block (obscuring ST-segment analysis) and history suggesting acute MI should also receive fibrinolytics or angioplasty.

Treatment Recommendations for AMI

Supportive Care for Chest Pain
- All patients should receive supplemental oxygen, 2 L/min by nasal canula, for a minimum of three hours
- Two large-bore IVs should be placed

Aspirin:

Inclusion	Clinical symptoms or suspicion of AMI
Exclusion	Aspirin allergy, active GI bleeding
Recommendation	Chew and swallow one dose of160-325 mg, then orally qd

Thrombolytics:

Inclusion	All patients with ischemic pain and ST-segment elevation (≥ 1 mm in ≥2 contiguous leads) within 12 hours of onset of persistent pain, age <75 years. All patients with a new bundle branch block and history suggesting acute MI.
Exclusion	Active internal bleeding; history of cerebrovascular accident; recent intracranial or intraspinal surgery or trauma; intracranial neoplasm, arteriovenous malformation, or aneurysm; known bleeding diathesis; severe uncontrolled hypertension
Recommendation	**Reteplase (Retavase)** 10 U IVP over 2 min x 2. Give second dose of 10 U 30 min after first dose **OR** **Tenecteplase (TNKase):** <60 kg: 30 mg IVP; 60-69 kg: 35 mg IVP; 70-79 kg: 40 mg IVP; 80-89 kg: 45 mg IVP; ≥90 kg: 50 mg IVP **OR** **t-PA (Alteplase, Activase)** 15 mg IV over 2 minutes, then 0.75 mg/kg (max 50 mg) IV over 30 min, followed by 0.5 mg/kg (max 35 mg) IV over 30 min.

Heparin:

Inclusion	**Administer concurrently with thrombolysis**
Exclusion	Active internal or CNS bleeding
Recommendation	Heparin 60 U/kg IVP, followed by 12 U/kg/hr continuous IV infusion x 48 hours. Maintain aPTT 50-70 seconds

Beta-Blockade:	
Inclusion	All patients with the diagnosis of AMI. Within 12 hours of diagnosis of AMI
Exclusion	Severe COPD, hypotension, bradycardia, AV block, pulmonary edema, cardiogenic shock
Recommendation	Metoprolol (Lopressor), 5 mg IV push every 5 minutes for three doses; followed by 25 mg PO bid. Titrate up to 100 mg PO bid **OR** Atenolol (Tenormin), 5 mg IV, repeated in 5 minutes, followed by 50-100 mg PO qd.
Nitrates:	
Inclusion	All patients with ischemic-type chest pain
Exclusion	Nitrate allergy; sildenafil (Viagra) within prior 24 hours; hypotension; caution in right ventricular infarction
Recommendation	0.4 mg NTG initially q 5 minutes, up to 3 doses or nitroglycerine aerosol, 1 spray sublingually every 5 minutes. IV infusion of NTG at 10-20 mcg/min, titrating upward by 5-10 mcg/min q 5-10 minutes (max 3 mcg/kg/min). Slow or stop infusion if systolic BP <90 mm Hg
ACE Inhibitors:	
Inclusion	All patients with the diagnosis of AMI. Initiate treatment within 24 hours after AMI
Exclusion	Bilateral renal artery stenosis, angioedema caused by previous treatment
Recommendation	Lisinopril (Prinivil) 2.5-5 mg qd, titrate to 10-20 mg qd. Maintain systolic BP >100 mm hg

C. Thrombolytics

   1. **ECG criteria for thrombolysis**
      a. ST Elevation (>1 mm in two or more contiguous leads), time to therapy 12 hours or less, age younger than 75 years.
      b. A new bundle branch block (obscuring ST-segment analysis) and history suggesting acute MI.
   2. **Alteplase (t-PA, tissue-plasminogen activator, Activase) and Reteplase (Retavase)** convert plasminogen to plasmin. Both agents are clot-specific and bind to new thrombus. Activase is superior to streptokinase. The alteplase thirty-day mortality rate of 6.3% is the lowest of the fibrinolytics, compared with 7.3% for streptokinase. Alteplase provides the earliest and most complete reperfusion.
   3. **Streptokinase (SK, Streptase)** provides greater benefit in older patients with a smaller amount of myocardium at risk who present later and those with a greater risk of ICH. The dose of IV SK is 1.5 million units given over 60 minutes.

D. Reperfusion therapy: Percutaneous coronary intervention

   1. PCI is preferable to thrombolytic therapy if performed in a timely fashion by individuals skilled in the procedure. Coronary angioplasty

provides higher rates of flow than thrombolytics and is associated with lower rates of reocclusion and postinfarction ischemia than fibrinolytic therapy.

2. Patients at high risk for mortality or severe LV dysfunction with signs of shock, pulmonary congestion, heart rate >100 bpm, and SBP <100 mm Hg should be sent to facilities capable of performing cardiac catheterization and rapid revascularization. When available within 90 minutes, PCI is recommended for all patients, particularly those who have a high risk of bleeding with fibrinolytic therapy.

E. **Heparin** is recommended in patients receiving selective fibrinolytic agents (tPA/Reteplase/tenectaplase). A bolus dose of 60 U/kg should be followed by infusion at a rate of 12 U/kg/hour (a maximum bolus of 4000 U/kg and infusion of 1000 U/h for patients weighing <70 kg). An aPTT of 50 to 70 seconds is optimal.

F. **Beta-blockade** use during and after AMI reduces mortality by 36%. Contraindications to beta-blockers include severe LV failure and pulmonary edema, bradycardia (heart rate <60 bpm), hypotension (SBP <100 mm Hg), signs of poor peripheral perfusion, second- or third-degree heart block.

1. **Metoprolol (Lopressor),** 5 mg IV push every 5 minutes for three doses; followed by 25 mg PO bid. Titrate up to 100 mg PO bid **OR**

2. **Atenolol (Tenormin),** 5 mg IV, repeated in 5 minutes, followed by 50-100 mg PO qd.

G. **ACE-inhibitors** increase survival in patients with AMI. ACE-inhibitors should be started between 6 to 24 hours after AMI and continued for 4-6 weeks, and indefinitely if ejection fraction <40%.

1. **Captopril (Capoten)** is given as a 6.25 mg initial dose and titrated up to 50 mg po bid, or

2. **Lisinopril (Prinivil)** may be given as 2.5-5 mg qd, titrate to 10-20 mg qd.

VI. **Management Non–Q-wave MI and high-risk unstable angina with ST-segment depression.**

A. **Non–Q-wave MI and unstable angina** present with ST-segment depression. Among patients with ST-segment depression, fibrinolytic therapy provides no benefit. Fibrinolytic therapy should not be used in patients with ST-segment depression or nondiagnostic ECGs.

B. **Aspirin** (325 mg qd) and **heparin**, 60 U/kg IVP, followed by 12 U/kg/hr continuous IV infusion x 48 hours (aPTT 50-70 seconds) should be given to patients with ST-segment depression or T-wave inversion with ischemic-type chest pain.

Heparin and ST-Segment Depression and Non–Q-Wave MI/Unstable Angina

- IV heparin therapy for 3 to 5 days is standard for high-risk and some intermediate-risk patients. Treat for 48 hours, then individualized therapy.
- LMWH is an acceptable alternative to IV unfractionated heparin.
  -Enoxaparin (Lovenox) 1.0 mg/kg SQ q12h **OR**
  -Dalteparin (Fragmin) 120 IU/kg (max 10,000 U) SQ q12h.

C. **Nitrates** should be given for recurrent angina. Sublingual nitroglycerin (NTG), initially, give up to three doses of 0.4 mg sublingual NTG every five minutes or nitroglycerine aerosol, 1 spray sublingually every 5 minutes. Nitroglycerin patch 0.2 mg/hr qd. Allow for nitrate-free period to prevent tachyphylaxis. Isosorbide dinitrate (Isordil) 10-60 mg PO tid [5,10,20, 30,40 mg], or isosorbide mononitrate (Imdur) 30-60 mg qd.

D. **Beta-blockers.** A beta-blocker should be initiated for patients with ST-segment depression.

1. Beta-blockers reduce the size of the infarct in patients who do not receive fibrinolytic therapy. A significant decrease in death and nonfatal infarction has been observed in patients treated with beta-blockers after infarction. Contraindications to beta-blockers: severe LV failure and pulmonary edema, bradycardia (heart rate <60 bpm), hypotension (SBP <100 mm Hg), signs of poor peripheral perfusion, second- or third-degree heart block.

2. **Metoprolol (Lopressor)**, 5 mg IV push every 5 minutes for three doses; followed by 25 mg PO bid. Titrate up to 100 mg PO **OR**

3. **Atenolol (Tenormin)**, 5 mg IV, repeated in 5 minutes, followed by 50-100 mg PO qd.

E. **Coronary angiography** is recommended for high-risk patients with recurrent ischemia, depressed LV function, widespread changes on the ECG, or prior MI.

F. **Glycoprotein IIb/IIIa inhibitors**

1. The GP IIb/IIIa receptor blockers reduce platelet aggregation. The GP IIb/IIIa inhibitors should be used for patients with non-ST-segment elevation MI or high-risk unstable angina. These agents should be used with aspirin or clopidogrel and unfractionated heparin. The dose of unfractionated heparin should be reduced by ⅓ when combined with GP blockers.

2. **Intravenous GP blocker dosages**

a. **Abciximab (ReoPro)**, 0.25 mg/kg IVP over 2 min, then 0.125 mcg/kg/min (max 10 mcg/min) for 12 hours.

b. **Eptifibatide (Integrilin)**, 180 mcg/kg IVP over 2 min, then 2 mcg/kg/min for 24-72 hours. Use 0.5 mcg/kg/min if creatinine is >2.0 mg/dL.

c. **Tirofiban (Aggrastat)**, 0.4 mcg/kg/min for 30 min, then 0.1 mcg/kg/min IV infusion for 24-72 hours. Reduce dosage by 50% if the creatine clearance is <30 mL/min.

VII. **Management of patients with a nondiagnostic ECG**

A. Patients with a nondiagnostic ECG who have an indeterminate or a low risk of MI should receive aspirin while undergoing serial cardiac enzyme studies and repeat ECGs.

B. Treadmill stress testing should be considered for patients with a suspicion of coronary ischemia.

Heart Failure

Congestive heart failure (CHF) is defined as the inability of the heart to meet the metabolic and nutritional demands of the body. Approximately 75% of patients with heart failure are older than 65-70 years of age. Approximately 8% of patients between the ages of 75 and 86 have heart failure.

I. Etiology
- **A.** The most common causes of CHF are coronary artery disease, hypertension, and alcoholic cardiomyopathy. Valvular diseases such as aortic stenosis and mitral regurgitation, are also common.
- **B.** Coronary artery disease is the etiology of heart failure in two-thirds of patients with left ventricular dysfunction. Heart failure should be presumed to be of ischemic origin until proven otherwise.

II. Clinical presentation
- **A.** Left heart failure produces dyspnea and fatigue. Right heart failure leads to lower extremity edema, ascites, congestive hepatomegaly, and jugular venous distension. Symptoms of pulmonary congestion include dyspnea, orthopnea, and paroxysmal nocturnal dyspnea. Clinical impairment is caused by left ventricular systolic dysfunction (ejection fraction of less than 40%) in 80-90% of patients with CHF.
- **B.** Patients should be evaluated for coronary artery disease, hypertension, and valvular dysfunction. Use of alcohol, chemotherapeutic agents (daunorubicin), negative inotropic agents, and symptoms of a recent viral syndrome should be assessed.
- **C.** CHF can present with shortness of breath, dyspnea on exertion, paroxysmal nocturnal dyspnea, orthopnea, nocturia, and cough. Exertional dyspnea is extremely common in patients with heart failure.

Precipitants of Congestive Heart Failure	
• Myocardial ischemia or infarction	• Thyroid disease
• Atrial fibrillation	• Pregnancy
• Worsening valvular disease	• Anemia
• Pulmonary embolism	• Infection
• Hypoxia	• Tachycardia or bradycardia
• Severe, uncontrolled hypertension	• Alcohol abuse
	• Medication or dietary noncompliance

- **D. Physical examination.** Lid lag, goiter, medication use, murmurs, abnormal heart rhythms may suggest a treatable underlying disease. Patients with CHF may present with resting tachycardia, jugular venous distension, a third heart sound, rales, lower extremity edema, or a laterally displaced apical impulse. Poor capillary refill, cool extremities, or an altered level of consciousness may also be present.

New York Heart Association Criteria for Heart Failure

Class I	Asymptomatic
Class II	Symptoms with moderate activity
Class III	Symptoms with minimal activity
Class IV	Symptoms at rest

- **E. Laboratory assessment**
  1. Patients with symptoms suggestive of CHF should have a 12-lead ECG.
  2. Impedance cardiography (ICG) is a noninvasive, reliable method of measuring cardiac index and stroke volume. It should be done on the first day of hospitalization and repeated to assess response to drug therapy.
  3. A chest x-ray should be performed to identify pleural effusions, pneumothorax, pulmonary edema, or infiltrates.
  4. If cardiac ischemia or infarction is suspected, cardiac enzymes should be drawn. A complete blood count, electrolytes, and digoxin level, if applicable, also are mandatory. Patients with suspected hyperthyroidism should have thyroid function studies drawn.
- **F. Echocardiography** is recommended to evaluate the presence of pericardial effusion, tamponade, valvular regurgitation, wall motion abnormalities, and ejection fraction.

Laboratory Workup for Suspected Heart Failure

Blood urea nitrogen	Magnesium
Cardiac enzymes (CK-MB, troponin, or both)	Thyroid-stimulating hormone
Complete blood cell count	Urinalysis
Creatinine	Echocardiogram
Electrolytes	Electrocardiography
Liver function tests	Impedance cardiography

III. Management of chronic heart failure
- **A.** Patients should also be placed on oxygen to maintain adequate oxygen saturation. In patients with severe symptoms (ie, pulmonary edema), continuous positive airway pressure (CPAP) or endotracheal intubation (ETI) may be employed.
- **B. Angiotensin-converting enzyme inhibitors** significantly reduce morbidity and mortality in CHF. Side effects include cough, worsening renal function, hyperkalemia, hypotension, and the risk of angioedema. ACEIs should be started at a very low dose and titrated up gradually to relieve shortness of breath. Renal function and electrolytes should be monitored.

ACE Inhibitors Used for Heart Failure

Benazepril (Lotensin) – start 10 mg po bid, target 20-40 mg po bid
Captopril (Capoten) – start 6.25-12.5 mg po tid, target dose 50-100 mg tid
Enalapril (Vasotec) – start 2.5 mg po qd/bid, target 2.5-10 mg tid
Fosinopril (Monopril) – start 10 mg po qd, target 20-40 mg/d
Lisinopril (Prinivil, Zestril) – start 5 mg po qd, target 5-20 mg/d
Quinapril (Accupril) – start 5 mg po bid, target 20-40 mg/d
Ramipril (Altace) – start 2.5 mg po bid, target 10 mg/d
Trandolapril (Mavik) – start 1 mg po qd, target 2-4 mg qd

C. **Angiotensin II receptor blockers (ARBs).** In patients who cannot tolerate or have contraindications to ACE inhibitors, ARBs should be considered. ARBs are as effective as ACE inhibitors with a lower incidence of cough and angioedema.

Angiotensin II Receptor Blockers for Heart Failure

Candesartan (Atacand) – start 4-8 mg qd bid, target 8-16 mg qd bid
Irbesartan (Avapro) – start 75-150 mg qd, target 150-300 mg qd
Losartan (Cozaar) – start 25-50 mg qd, target 50 mg bid
Valsartan (Diovan) – start 80 mg qd, target 160-320 mg qd

D. **Hydralazine/Isordil combination** may be used in patients who are intolerant to ACE-inhibitors and ARBs; however, this combination is less effective in reducing mortality. Hydralazine can cause reflex tachycardia and increase ischemic pain. Reflex tachycardia due to hydralazine may be beneficial in patients with bradycardia caused by beta-blockers. The dosage of hydralazine is 10-50 mg qid, combined with isosorbide dinitrate (Isordil) 10-40 mg qid, OR isordil mononitrate (Imdur) 30-60 mg qd.

E. **Diuretics** induce peripheral vasodilation, reduce cardiac filling pressures, and prevent fluid retention. Loop diuretics are the most potent agents in CHF. Diuretics should be prescribed for patients with heart failure who have volume overload.

Diuretic Therapy in Congestive Heart Failure

Loop diuretics
- Furosemide (Lasix) – 20-200 mg IV/PO daily or bid, or 10-20 mg/hr IV infusion
- Bumetanide (Bumex) – 0.5-4.0 mg IV/PO daily or bid
- Torsemide (Demadex) – 5-100 mg IV/PO daily

Long-acting thiazide diuretics
- Metolazone (Zaroxolyn) – 2.5-10.0 mg qd PO bid
- Hydrochlorothiazide – 25 PO mg qd

Aldosterone Antagonists
- Spironolactone (Aldactone) 12.5-25 mg PO qd

F. **Beta-Blockers** are beneficial in heart failure, improving contractility and survival. Beta-blockers should be started at low doses and advanced slowly. Beta-blockers should not be used in acute pulmonary edema or decompensated heart failure, and they should only be initiated in the stable patient. Beta-blockers are an add-on therapy for patients being treated with ACE inhibitors.

Carvedilol, Metoprolol, and Bisoprolol – Dosages and Side Effects

- Carvedilol (Coreg) – start at 1.625-3.125 mg bid; target dose 25-50 mg bid
- Metoprolol (Lopressor) – start at 12.5 mg bid; target dose 100 mg bid
- Bisoprolol (Zebeta) – start at 1.25 mg qd; target dose 10 mg qd

---

Digoxin Dosing

- Start at 0.250 mg/d with near normal renal function; start at 0.125 mg/d if renal function impaired.
- Maintain serum digoxin level of 0.8-1.2 ng/mL.

- **G. Digoxin** does not improve survival in CHF (as do ACE-inhibitors and beta-blockers). Digoxin may be added to a regimen of ACE-inhibitors and diuretics if symptoms of heart failure persist. Digoxin can increase exercise tolerance, improve symptoms, and decrease the risk of hospitalization.
- **H. Spironolactone** improves mortality in severe CHF and should be used in addition to an ACE-inhibitor or ARB. A dosage of 25 mg qd should be considered in patients with severe CHF. It can cause hyperkalemia, rash, and gynecomastia.
- **I. Nonpharmacologic treatments**
  1. Salt restriction (a diet with 2 g sodium or less), alcohol restriction, water restriction for patients with severe renal impairment, and regular aerobic exercise as tolerated.
  2. Synchronized biventricular pacing in patients with an ejection fraction of <40% and wide QRS duration of >150 msec may improve symptoms and the overall clinical course.
- **J. Inotropic support**
  1. Positive inotropic agents improve quality of life and reduce need for hospitalization but increase mortality. Parenterally positive inotropic therapy increases cardiac output and decreases symptoms of congestion.
  2. Parenteral inotropic agents can be administered continuously in patients with exacerbations of heart failure. These agents may be administered continuously or intermittently at home. Impedance cardiography is used to assess clinical response before and during treatment.

Inotropic Agents for Cardiogenic Shock

- Milrinone (Primacor) – start at 0.375 mcg/kg/min and titrate to 0.75 mcg/kg/min
- Dobutamine (Dobutrex) – start at 2-3 mcg/kg/min and titrate 5 mcg/kg/min
- Dopamine (Intropin) – start at 2-5 mcg/kg/min and titrate to 10 mcg/kg/min

---

  K. Natriuretic peptides
    1. Atrial and brain natriuretic peptides regulate cardiovascular homeostasis and fluid volume.
    2. Nesiritide (Natrecor) is structurally similar to atrial natriuretic peptide. It has natriuretic, diuretic, vasodilatory, smooth-muscle relaxant properties, and inhibits the renin-angiotensin system. Nesiritide is indicated for the treatment of moderate-to-severe heart failure.
    3. The initial dose of nesiritide is 0.015 mcg/kg/min IV infusion slowly titrated to max 0.03 mcg/kg/min. Hypotension occurs frequently with a mild increase in heart rate.

Treatment of Acute Heart Failure/Pulmonary Edema

- Oxygen therapy, 2 L/min by nasal canula
- Furosemide (Lasix) 20-80 mg IV (patients already on outpatient dose may require more)
- Nitroglycerine start at 10-20 mcg/min and titrate to BP (use with caution if inferior/right ventricular infarction suspected)
- Sublingual nitroglycerin 0.4 mg
- Morphine sulfate 2-4 mg IV. Avoid if inferior wall MI suspected or if hypotensive or presence of tenuous airway
- Potassium supplementation prn

Atrial Fibrillation

Atrial fibrillation (AF) is the most common arrhythmia. The median age of onset is 75, and the incidence and prevalence increase dramatically with age. For patients older than 80 years, the incidence of AF is 9%. For patients aged 80-90, nearly one-third of strokes that occur are related to AF.

I. Pathophysiology. The cardiac conditions most commonly associated with AF are coronary artery disease, hypertension, rheumatic heart disease, mitral valve disease, cardiomyopathies, and open-heart surgery. Hypertension and coronary artery disease are the most frequent risk factors, accounting for 65% of AF cases. The most common noncardiac causes are pulmonary diseases (including COPD), hypoxia, and hyperthyroidism.

II. Clinical evaluation
  A. Patients with AF often experience dyspnea and palpitations, although some may be asymptomatic. AF may be associated with palpitations, dizziness, dyspnea, chest pain, syncope, fatigue, or confusion.

B. The most common physical sign of AF is an irregular pulse. Other physical exam findings include a pulse deficit, absent "a" wave in the jugular venous pulse, and a variable intensity of the first heart sound.

Causes of Atrial Fibrillation

Structural Heart Disease	Absence of Structural Heart Disease
Hypertension	Pulmonary diseases: COPD, hypoxia,
Ischemic heart disease	pneumonia, pulmonary embolus,
Valvular heart disease: Mitral stenosis,	metabolic disorders, thyrotoxicosis,
aortic stenosis, mitral regurgitation	electrolyte imbalance
Pericarditis	Acute ethanol intoxication
Cardiac tumors	Methylxanthine derivatives:
Sick sinus syndrome	Theophylline, caffeine
Cardiomyopathies	Systemic illness Sepsis, malignancy
Congenital heart disease	Lone atrial fibrillation
Wolf-Parkinson-White syndrome	

III. Diagnostic studies

A. Laboratory studies should include chemistries, CBC, INR/PTT, and a TSH. A chest x-ray may uncover COPD, pneumonia, CHF, or cardiomegaly.

B. Ambulatory 24-hour (Holter) ECG monitoring should be performed to determine both the frequency and duration of AF.

C. Echocardiogram provides information on cardiac dimensions (left atrial size), LV systolic function, valvular disease, and LV hypertrophy.

IV. Initial management

A. If the duration of AF is less than 48 hours, the initial goals are either cardioversion or ventricular rate control and observation. If the patient is not hemodynamically compromised and the AF is of new onset, an initial period of observation using medications for rate control and anticoagulation with heparin are initiated. If AF persists despite rate control, restoration of sinus rhythm is the usual goal if the patient is symptomatic during AF, requires AV synchrony for improved cardiac output, or wants to avoid lifelong anticoagulation. Sinus rhythm can be achieved with either external cardioversion and/or pharmacological agents.

B. Initial treatment of atrial fibrillation

1. Anticoagulation in patients with nonvalvular AF reduces the incidence of embolic strokes.

2. Oral anticoagulation therapy with warfarin (Coumadin), with an INR goal between 2.0-3.0, should be considered in all AF patients with one or more risk factors, as described below, regardless of age.

3. In patients without rheumatic heart disease who are younger than 75 years of age, warfarin therapy should be initiated if risk factors are present, including previous transient ischemic attack or stroke, hypertension, heart failure, diabetes, clinical coronary artery disease, mitral stenosis, prosthetic heart valves, or thyrotoxicosis. In patients younger than 65 and without these risk factors (lone AF), aspirin alone may be appropriate for stroke prevention.

4. Patients between the ages of 65 and 75 with none of these risk factors could be treated with either warfarin or aspirin.

5. In patients older than 75 with AF, oral anticoagulation with warfarin is recommended. In patients with major contraindications to warfarin (intracranial hemorrhage, unstable gait, falls, syncope, or poor compliance), a daily aspirin is a reasonable alternative.

6. If the duration of AF is unknown or more than 48 hours, then rate control and anticoagulation therapy should be initiated first. The patient should be evaluated for the presence of an intracardiac thrombus with a transesophageal echocardiography (TEE). If the TEE demonstrates a clot, the patient is anticoagulated for three weeks before a scheduled cardioversion. If no left atrial thrombus is identified by TEE, heparin is started and the patient is cardioverted. Following successful cardioversion, the patient is placed on warfarin for an additional four weeks.

C. Rate control

1. Patients with AF of greater than one year duration or a left atrial size greater than 50 mm may have difficulty in converting to sinus rhythm. In these patients, rate control, rather than conversion to sinus rhythm may, be beneficial. A controlled ventricular rate in AF is less than 90 bpm at rest.

2. The pharmacological agents used for rate control are calcium channel blockers (diltiazem, verapamil), beta-blockers (metoprolol, esmolol) and digoxin. Calcium channel blockers should be used first because of rapid onset of action compared to digoxin, which takes 4-6 hours to show pharmacological effect. Digoxin is the first drug of choice in significant left ventricular dysfunction.

3. **Calcium channel blockers** can slow AV node conduction and are first-line agents for rate control therapy.

4. **Beta-blockers** slow AV nodal and sinoatrial nodal conduction. The most commonly used beta-blockers are metoprolol and atenolol.

5. **Digoxin** has numerous drug interactions, an unpredictable dose response curve, and a potentially lethal toxicity. Digoxin is is reserved for patients with systolic dysfunction and heart failure.

Agents Used for Heart Rate Control in Atrial Fibrillation

Agent	Loading Dose	Onset of Action	Maintenance Dosage	Major Side Effects
Diltiazem (Cardizem)	0.25 mg per kg IV over 2 minutes, may repeat dose with 0.35 mg/kg after 15 min x 1	2-7 minutes	5-15 mg per hour IV or 120-360 mg PO every day in divided doses	Hypotension, heart block, heart failure
Verapamil (Calan, Isoptin)	0.075-0.15 mg per kg IV over 2 minutes	3-5 minutes	240-360 mg PO every day in divided doses	Hypotension, heart block, heart failure

Agent	Loading Dose	Onset of Action	Maintenance Dosage	Major Side Effects
Esmolol (Brevibloc)	0.5 mg per kg IV over one minute	5 minutes	0.05-0.2 mg/kg/minute IV	Hypotension, heart block, bradycardia, asthma, heart failure
Metoprolol (Lopressor)	2.5-5 mg IV bolus over 2 minutes, up to 3 doses	5 minutes	50-200 mg PO every day in 2 daily doses	Hypotension, heart block, bradycardia, asthma, heart failure
Propranolol (Inderal)	0.15 mg per kg	5 minutes	40-320 mg PO every day in divided doses	Hypotension, heart block, bradycardia, asthma, heart failure
Digoxin (Lanoxin)	0.25 mg IV or PO every 4 hours, up to 1.0-1.5 mg	4-6 hours	0.125-0.25 mg PO/IV qd	Digitalis toxicity, heart block, bradycardia, ventricular fibrillation

Agents Used for Heart Rate Control in Atrial Fibrillation				
Drug	Mechanism of Action	ECG Changes	Dose	Adverse Reaction
Class la Agents				
Quinidine	Decrease Na influx Reduce upstroke velocity. Prolong repolarization	QRS widens, QT lengthens	Sulfate 300-600 mg po q6-8hrs Quinaglute 324-628 mg po q8-12 hrs	GI, cinchonism VT/VF/ Torsade de Pointes
Procainamide		QRS widens, QT lengthens	Load: IV 13-17 mg/kg over 30-60 min Maintenance: IV 2-4 mg/min or Procan SR 750-1500 mg po q6hr	SLE-like syndrome, confusion

Class Ic Agents				
Flecainide	Reduction in upstroke velocity	QRS widens, QT lengthens	Start 50-100 mg po q12hr; max. 200 bid	Dizziness, headaches
Propafenone		QRS widens, QT lengthens	Start 150 mg po q8hrs; max. 300 mg po q8hr	Dry mouth, GI, dizziness
Class III Agents				
Amiodarone	Blocks K efflux, prolongs repolarization	Dose-dependant QT prolongation	Load 400 mg po tid x 7-14 days, then 400 mg po qd x 1 month; Maintenance: 100-400 mg/day	Ataxia, tremors pulmonary fibrosis, pneumonitis/alveolitis, skin discoloration, thyroid and LFT abnormalities
Sotalol	Potent beta-blocking activity		80 mg po bid; max. 160 mg bid	Bradycardia, Torsade de Pointes.
Ibutilide	Prolong action potential and refractory period		1 mg IV infusion over 10 min, may repeat once after 10 min	Torsade in 3-8%
Dofetilide			125-500 mcg bid, depending on renal function	0.5-10% torsade

D. **Antiarrhythmics.** Restoration of sinus rhythm is the optimal goal, as it may relieve symptoms and improve cardiac output.
  1. **Class Ia.** These medications act by blocking the fast sodium channel, reducing the impulse conduction through the myocardium.
    a. **Quinidine** can be used for acute conversion as well as to maintain of sinus rhythm.
    b. **Procainamide** can also be used for both acute conversion and maintenance. It is slightly less effective than quinidine.
    c. **Disopyramide** has negative inotropic properties. Disopyramide is infrequently used in the treatment of AF due to poor efficacy and frequent side effects.
  2. **Class Ic.** This class of medications acts by prolonging intraventricular conduction.
    a. **Flecainide** can cause acute conversion to sinus rhythm in 50-55%. Due to its negative inotropic action, flecainide should be used cautiously in patients with AF and hypertrophic cardiomyopathy. It should not be used in patients with structural heart disease. It is reserved for patients with normal LV function and refractory AF.

b. **Propafenone** may have fewer side effects and is better tolerated than the Ia agents. It is available only in an oral form and can also be given as a single bolus dose for AF of less than 24 hours. Proarrhythmia can occur but is reported less frequently than with the other Ic medications. Propafenone is useful for patients who are hypertensive and have a structurally normal heart with AF. Propafenone should be avoided in patients with structural heart disease.

3. **Class III.** The medications in this class act by blocking outward potassium currents, resulting in increased myocardial refractoriness. All class III agents cause a dose-dependent QTc prolongation, resulting in Torsades de Pointes. These agents are contraindicated if the QTc is >0.44 seconds.

   a. **Amiodarone (Cordarone)** has sodium, calcium, and beta-blocking effects. Amiodarone has a low proarrhythmia profile. It is safe and efficacious in patients with CHF and AF. Side effects include pulmonary fibrosis, pneumonitis, skin discoloration, thyroid and liver abnormalities, ataxia, and tremors (33%).

   b. **Sotalol (Betapace)** has a beta-blocking effect. It is less effective than quinidine, with a conversion rate of 20%. It is most appropriate for sinus maintenance in patients with AF and coronary artery disease. Sotalol should be avoided in patients with severe LV dysfunction and COPD.

   c. **Ibutilide (Corvert)** is highly effective for the conversion of recent onset AF (30%) and atrial flutter (70%). Polymorphic ventricular tachycardia occurs in about 6%. Pretreatment with magnesium may prevent polymorphic ventricular tachycardia.

   d. **Dofetilide (Tikosyn)** is indicated for acute conversion and maintenance of atrial fibrillation. The success rate in acute conversion is 30%.

E. **Nonpharmacologic strategies.** Due to drug intolerance, possible proarrhythmic effects, and disappointing long-term efficacy of the antiarrhythmic agents, non-pharmacological therapies have an important role in the management of AF.

   1. **Electrical cardioversion** is rapid and highly effective, with success rates greater than 80%.

   2. **Radiofrequency catheter ablation/atrial defibrillators.** The delivery of radiofrequency current through a catheter tip advanced to the atrium is highly effective and safe.

Hypertensive Emergency

Hypertensive crises are severe elevations in blood pressure (BP) characterized by a diastolic blood pressure (BP) higher than 120-130 mm Hg.

I. **Clinical evaluation of hypertensive crises**

A. **Hypertensive emergency** is defined by a diastolic blood pressure >120 mm Hg associated with ongoing vascular damage. Symptoms or signs of neurologic, cardiac, renal, or retinal dysfunction are present. Hypertensive emergencies include severe hypertension in the following settings:

   1. Aortic dissection

2. Acute left ventricular failure and pulmonary edema
3. Acute renal failure or worsening of chronic renal failure
4. Hypertensive encephalopathy
5. Focal neurologic damage indicating thrombotic or hemorrhagic stroke
6. Pheochromocytoma, cocaine overdose, or other hyperadrenergic states
7. Unstable angina or myocardial infarction
8. Eclampsia

B. **Hypertensive urgency** is defined as diastolic blood pressure >120 mm Hg without evidence of vascular damage; the disorder is asymptomatic and no retinal lesions are present.

C. **Causes of secondary hypertension** include renovascular hypertension, pheochromocytoma, cocaine use, withdrawal from alpha-2 stimulants, clonidine, beta-blockers or alcohol, and noncompliance with antihypertensive medications.

II. Initial assessment of severe hypertension

A. When severe hypertension is noted, the measurement should be repeated in both arms to detect any significant differences. Peripheral pulses should be assessed for absence or delay, which suggests dissecting aortic dissection. Evidence of pulmonary edema should be sought.

B. Target organ damage is suggested by chest pain, neurologic signs, altered mental status, profound headache, dyspnea, abdominal pain, hematuria, focal neurologic signs (paralysis or paresthesia), or hypertensive retinopathy.

C. Prescription drug use should be assessed, including missed doses of antihypertensives. History of recent cocaine or amphetamine use should be sought.

D. If focal neurologic signs are present, a CT scan may be required to differentiate hypertensive encephalopathy from a stroke syndrome.

III. Laboratory evaluation

A. Complete blood cell count, urinalysis for protein, glucose, and blood; urine sediment examination; chemistry panel (SMA-18).

B. If chest pain is present, cardiac enzymes are obtained.

C. If the history suggests a hyperadrenergic state, the possibility of a pheochromocytoma should be excluded with a 24-hour urine for catecholamines. A urine drug screen may be necessary to exclude illicit drug use.

D. Electrocardiogram should be completed.

E. Suspected primary aldosteronism can be excluded with a 24-hour urine potassium and an assessment of plasma renin activity. Renal artery stenosis can be excluded with captopril renography and intravenous pyelography.

Screening Tests for Secondary Hypertension	
Renovascular Hypertension	Captopril renography: Renal scan before and after 25 mg PO Intravenous pyelography MRI angiography

Hyperaldosteronism	Serum potassium 24-hr urine potassium Plasma renin activity CT scan of adrenals
Pheochromocytoma	24-hr urine catecholamines CT scan Nuclear MIBG scan
Cushing's Syndrome	Plasma ACTH Dexamethasone suppression test
Hyperparathyroidism	Serum calcium Serum parathyroid hormone

IV. Management of hypertensive emergencies

A. The patient should be hospitalized for intravenous access, continuous intra-arterial blood pressure monitoring, and electrocardiographic monitoring. Volume status and urinary output should be monitored. Rapid, uncontrolled reductions in blood pressure should be avoided because coma, stroke, myocardial infarction, acute renal failure, or death may result.

B. The goal of initial therapy is to terminate ongoing target organ damage. The mean arterial pressure should be lowered not more than 20-25%, or to a diastolic blood pressure of 100 mm Hg over 15 to 30 minutes.

V. Parenteral antihypertensive agents

A. Nitroprusside (Nipride)

1. Nitroprusside is the drug of choice in almost all hypertensive emergencies (except myocardial ischemia or renal impairment). It dilates both arteries and veins, and it reduces afterload and preload. Onset of action is nearly instantaneous, and the effects disappear 1-2 minutes after discontinuation.

2. The starting dosage is 0.25-0.5 mcg/kg/min by continuous infusion with a range of 0.25-8.0 mcg/kg/min. Titrate dose to gradually reduce blood pressure over minutes to hours.

3. When treatment is prolonged or when renal insufficiency is present, the risk of cyanide and thiocyanate toxicity is increased. Signs of thiocyanate toxicity include anorexia, disorientation, fatigue, hallucinations, nausea, toxic psychosis, and seizures.

B. Nitroglycerin

1. Nitroglycerin is the drug of choice for hypertensive emergencies with coronary ischemia. It should not be used with hypertensive encephalopathy because it increases intracranial pressure.

2. Nitroglycerin increases venous capacitance, decreases venous return and left ventricular filling pressure. It has a rapid onset of action of 2-5 minutes. Tolerance may occur within 24-48 hours.

3. The starting dose is 15 mcg IV bolus, then 5-10 mcg/min (50 mg in 250 mL D5W). Titrate by increasing the dose at 3- to 5-minute intervals up to max 1.0 mcg/kg/min.

C. Labetalol IV (Normodyne)

1. Labetalol is a good choice if BP elevation is associated with hyperadrenergic activity, aortic dissection, an aneurysm, or postoperative hypertension.

2. Labetalol is administered as 20 mg slow IV over 2 min. Additional doses of 20-80 mg may be administered q5-10min, then q3-4h prn or 0.5-2.0 mg/min IV infusion. Labetalol is contraindicated in obstructive pulmonary disease, CHF, or heart block greater than first degree.

D. Enalaprilat IV (Vasotec)

1. Enalaprilat is an ACE-inhibitor with a rapid onset of action (15 min) and long duration of action (11 hours). It is ideal for patients with heart failure or accelerated-malignant hypertension.

2. Initial dose, 1.25 mg IVP (over 2-5 min) q6h, then increase up to 5 mg q6h. Reduce dose in azotemic patients. Contraindicated in bilateral renal artery stenosis.

E. Esmolol (Brevibloc) is a non-selective beta-blocker with a 1-2 min onset of action and short duration of 10 min. The dose is 500 mcg/kg/min x 1 min, then 50 mcg/kg/min; max 300 mcg/kg/min IV infusion.

F. Hydralazine is a preload and afterload reducing agent. It is ideal in hypertension due to eclampsia. Reflex tachycardia is common. The dose is 20 mg IV/IM q4-6h.

G. Nicardipine (Cardene IV) is a calcium channel blocker. It is contraindicated in presence of CHF. Tachycardia and headache are common. The onset of action is 10 min, and the duration is 2-4 hours. The dose is 5 mg/hr continuous infusion, up to 15 mg/hr.

H. Fenoldopam (Corlopam) is a vasodilator. It may cause reflex tachycardia and headaches. The onset of action is 2-3 min, and the duration is 30 min. The dose is 0.01 mcg/kg/min IV infustion titrated, up to 0.3 mcg/kg/min.

I. Phentolamine (Regitine) is an intravenous alpha-adrenergic antagonist used in excess catecholamine states, such as pheochromocytomas, rebound hypertension due to withdrawal of clonidine, and drug ingestions. The dose is 2-5 mg IV every 5 to 10 minutes.

J. Trimethaphan (Arfonad) is a ganglionic-blocking agent. It is useful in dissecting aortic aneurysm when beta-blockers are contraindicated; however, it is rarely used because most physicians are more familiar with nitroprusside. The dosage of trimethoprim is 0.3-3 mg/min IV infusion.

Ventricular Arrhythmias

I. Ventricular fibrillation and tachycardia

-If unstable (see ACLS protocol page 5), defibrillate with unsynchronized 200 J, 300 J, then 360 J.

-Oxygen 100% by mask.

-Procainamide loading dose 10-15 mg/kg at 20 mg/min IV or 100 mg IV q10min, then 2-4 mg/min IV maintenance **OR**

-**Also see "other antiarrhythmics" below.**

II. Torsades de Pointes

-Correct underlying cause and consider discontinuing drugs that cause Torsades de Pointes (dofetilide, ibutilide, sotalol, amiodarone, quinidine, procainamide, disopyramide, moricizine, bepridil, phenothiazines, tricyclic and tetracyclic antidepressants, vasopressin, imidazoles, pentamidine); correct hypokalemia and hypomagnesemia.

-Defibrillate with 360 J.

-Magnesium sulfate (drug of choice), 2 gm IV push.

-Isoproterenol (Isuprel) 2-20 µg/min (2 mg in 500 mL D5W, 4 µg/mL) **OR**
-Phenytoin (Dilantin) 100-300 mg IV given in 50 mg increments q5min.

III. Other antiarrhythmics
Class Ib
-Lidocaine 50-100 mg (1 mg/kg) IV, then 2-4 mg/min IV.
-Mexiletine (Mexitil) 100-200 mg PO q8h, max 1200 mg/d.
-Tocainide (Tonocard) loading 400-600 mg PO, then 400-600 mg PO q8-12h; max 1800 mg/d.
-Phenytoin (Dilantin), loading dose 15 mg/kg at 50 mg/min, then 100 IV q8h.

Class Ic
-Flecainide (Tambocor) 50-100 mg PO q12h, max 400 mg/d.
-Propafenone (Rythmol) 150-300 mg PO q8h, max 1200 mg/d.

Class III
-Amiodarone (Cordarone) PO loading 400-1200 mg/d in divided doses x 5-14 days, then 200-400 mg PO qd **OR** 150 mg slow IV over 10 min, then 1 mg/min IV infusion x 6 hours then 0.5 mg/min IV infusion thereafter.
-Sotalol (Betapace) 40-80 mg PO bid, max160 mg bid.
Labs: SMA 12, Mg, calcium, CBC, cardiac enzymes, LFTs, ABG, drug levels, thyroid function test. ECG, electrophysiologic study.

Acute Pericarditis

Pericarditis is the most common disease of the pericardium. The most common cause of pericarditis is viral infection. This disorder is characterized by chest pain, a pericardial friction rub, electrocardiographic changes, and pericardial effusion.

I. Clinical features
A. Chest pain of acute infectious (viral) pericarditis typically develops in younger adults 1 to 2 weeks after a "viral illness." The chest pain is of sudden and severe onset, with retrosternal and/or left precordial pain and referral to the back and trapezius ridge. Pain may be preceded by low-grade fever. Radiation to the arms may also occur. The pain is often pleuritic (eg, accentuated by inspiration or coughing) and may also be relieved by changes in posture (upright posture).
B. A pericardial friction rub is the most important physical sign. It is often described as triphasic, with systolic and both early (passive ventricular filling) and late (atrial systole) diastolic components, or more commonly a biphasic (systole and diastole).
C. Resting tachycardia (rarely atrial fibrillation) and a low-grade fever may be present.

Causes of Pericarditis	
Idiopathic	Hypersensitivity: drug
Infectious: Viral, bacterial, tuberculous, parasitic, fungal	Postmyocardial injury syndrome
	Trauma
Connective tissue diseases Metabolic: uremia, hypothyroidism Neoplasm, radiation	Dissecting aneurysm
	Chylopericardium

II. Diagnostic testing

A. **ECG changes.** During the initial few days, diffuse (limb leads and precordial leads) ST segment elevations are common in the absence of reciprocal ST segment depression. PR segment depression is also common and reflects atrial involvement.

B. The chest radiograph is often unrevealing, although a small left pleural effusion may be seen. An elevated erythrocyte sedimentation rate and C-reactive protein (CRP) and mild elevations of the white blood cell count are also common.

C. **Labs:** CBC, SMA 12, albumin, viral serologies: Coxsackie A & B, measles, mumps, influenza, ASO titer, hepatitis surface antigen, ANA, rheumatoid factor, anti-myocardial antibody, PPD with candida, mumps. Cardiac enzymes q8h x 4, ESR, blood C&S X 2.

D. **Pericardiocentesis:** Gram stain, C&S, cell count & differential, cytology, glucose, protein, LDH, amylase, triglyceride, AFB, specific gravity, pH.

E. **Echocardiography** is the most sensitive test for detecting pericardial effusion, which may occur with pericarditis.

III. Treatment of acute pericarditis (nonpurulent)

A. If effusion present on echocardiography, pericardiocentesis should be performed and the catheter should be left in place for drainage.

B. Treatment of pain starts with nonsteroidal anti-inflammatory drugs, meperidine, or morphine. In some instances, corticosteroids may be required to suppress inflammation and pain.

C. **Anti-inflammatory treatment with NSAIDs is first-line therapy.**
  1. Indomethacin (Indocin) 25 mg tid or 75 mg SR qd, **OR**
  2. Ketorolac (Toradol) 15-30 mg IV q6h, **OR**
  3. Ibuprofen (Motrin) 600 mg q8h.

D. **Morphine sulfate** 5-15 mg intramuscularly every 4-6 hours. Meperidine (Demerol) may also be used, 50-100 mg IM/IV q4-6h prn pain and promethazine (Phenergan) 25-75 mg IV q4h.

E. **Prednisone,** 60 mg daily, to be reduced every few days to 40, 20, 10, and 5 mg daily.

F. **Purulent pericarditis**
  1. Nafcillin or oxacillin 2 gm IV q4h **AND EITHER**
  2. Gentamicin or tobramycin 100-120 mg IV (1.5-2 mg/kg); then 80 mg (1.0-1.5 mg/kg) IV q8h (adjust in renal failure) **OR**
  3. Ceftizoxime (Cefizox) 1-2 gm IV q8h.
  4. Vancomycin, 1 gm IV q12h, may be used in place of nafcillin or oxacillin.

Pacemakers

Indications for implantation of a permanent pacemaker are based on symptoms, the presence of heart disease and the presence of symptomatic bradyarrhythmias. Pacemakers are categorized by a three- to five-letter code according to the site of the pacing electrode and the mode of pacing.

I. Indications for pacemakers

A. **First-degree atrioventricular (AV)** block can be associated with severe symptoms. Pacing may benefit patients with a PR interval greater than

0.3 seconds. Type I second-degree AV block does not usually require permanent pacing because progression to a higher degree AV block is not common. Permanent pacing improves survival in patients with complete heart block.

B. Permanent pacing is not needed in reversible causes of AV block, such as electrolyte disturbances or Lyme disease. Implantation is easier and of lower cost with single-chamber ventricular demand (VVI) pacemakers, but use of these devices is becoming less common with the advent of dual-chamber demand (DDD) pacemakers.

Generic Pacemaker Codes

Position 1 (chamber paced)	Position 2 (chamber sensed)	Position 3 (response to sensing)	Position 4 (programmable functions; rate modulation)	Position 5 (antitachyarrhythmia functions)
V--ventricle	V--ventricle	T--triggered	P--programmable rate and/or output	P--pacing (antitachyarrhythmia)
A--atrium	A--atrium	I--inhibited	M--multiprogrammability of rate, output, sensitivity, etc.	S--shock
D--dual (A & V)	D--dual (A & V)	D--dual (T & I)	C--communicating (telemetry)	D--dual (P + S)
O--none	O--none	O--none	R--rate modulation O--none	O--none

C. Sick sinus syndrome (or sinus node dysfunction) is the most common reason for permanent pacing. Symptoms are related to the bradyarrhythmias of sick sinus syndrome. VVI mode is typically used in patients with sick sinus syndrome, but recent studies have shown that DDD pacing improves morbidity, mortality and quality of life.

II. Temporary pacemakers

A. Temporary pacemaker leads generally are inserted percutaneously, then positioned in the right ventricular apex and attached to an external generator. Temporary pacing is used to stabilize patients awaiting permanent pacemaker implantation, to correct a transient symptomatic bradycardia due to drug toxicity or to suppress Torsades de Pointes by maintaining a rate of 85-100 beats per minute until the cause has been eliminated.

B. Temporary pacing may also be used in a prophylactic fashion in patients at risk of symptomatic bradycardia during a surgical procedure or high-degree AV block in the setting of an acute myocardial infarction.

C. In emergent situations, ventricular pacing can be instituted immediately by transcutaneous pacing using electrode pads applied to the chest wall.

References

ACC/AHA Guidelines for Management of Patients with Acute Myocardial Infarction. Circulation 1999; 100; 1016-1030.

ACC/AHA Guidelines for Management of Patients with Unstable Angina and NonST-Segment Elevation Myocardial Infarction. Circulation 2000; 102; 1193-1209.

Acute Coronary Syndromes (Acute Myocardial Infarction). Circulation 2000; 102 (supp I): I172-I203.

Consensus recommendations for the management of chronic heart failure. Am J Card (supp) Jan 21, 1999.

Bristow MR, et al: Heart failure management using implantable devices for ventricular resynchronization: Companion Trial. J of Cardiac Failure, 2000: 6; 276-284.

Yeghiazarians, Y. et al: Unstable Angina Pectoris: NEJM 2000; 342 #2; 101-112.

Wright, RS et al: Update on Intravenous Fibrinolytic Therapy for Acute Myocardial Infarction. Mayo Clin Proc 2000; 75:1185-92.

Adams, et al. Heart Failure Society Guidelines. Pharmacotherapy 2000; 20 (5): 496-520

Skrabal, et al. Advances in the Treatment of CHF: New Approaches for an Old Disease. Pharmacotherapy 2000; 20 (7): 787-804.

Pulmonary Disorders

T. Scott Gallacher, MD
Ryan Klein, MD
Michael Krutzik, MD
Thomas Vovan, MD

Orotracheal Intubation

Endotracheal Tube Size (interior diameter):
  Women 7.0-9.0 mm
  Men 8.0-10.0 mm

1. Prepare suction apparatus. Have Ambu bag and mask apparatus setup with 100% oxygen; and ensure that patient can be adequately bag ventilated and suction apparatus is available.
2. If sedation and/or paralysis is required, consider rapid sequence induction as follows:
   A. Fentanyl (Sublimaze) 50 mcg increments IV (1 mcg/kg) with:
   B. Midazolam (Versed) 1 mg IV q2-3 min. max 0.1-0.15 mg/kg followed by:
   C. Succinylcholine (Anectine) 0.6-1.0 mg/kg, at appropriate intervals; or vecuronium (Norcuron) 0.1 mg/kg IV x 1.
   D. Propofol (Diprivan): 0.5 mg/kg IV bolus.
   E. Etomidate (Amidate): 0.3-0.4 mg/kg IV.
3. Position the patient's head in the sniffing position with head flexed at neck and extended. If necessary, elevate the head with a small pillow.
4. Ventilate the patient with bag mask apparatus and hyperoxygenate with 100% oxygen.
5. Hold laryngoscope handle with left hand, and use right hand to open the patient's mouth. Insert blade along the right side of mouth to the base of tongue, and push the tongue to the left. If using curved blade, advance it to the vallecula (superior to epiglottis), and lift anteriorly, being careful not to exert pressure on the teeth. If using a straight blade, place beneath the epiglottis and lift anteriorly.
6. Place endotracheal tube (ETT) into right corner of mouth and pass it through the vocal cords; stop just after the cuff disappears behind vocal cords. If unsuccessful after 30 seconds, stop and resume bag and mask ventilation before re-attempting. A stilette to maintain the shape of the ETT in a hockey stick shape may be used. Remove stilette after intubation.
7. Inflate cuff with syringe keeping cuff pressure <20 cm H_2O, and attach the tube to an Ambu bag or ventilator. Confirm bilateral, equal expansion of the chest and equal bilateral breath sounds. Auscultate the abdomen to confirm that the ETT is not in the esophagus. If there is any question about proper ETT location, repeat laryngoscopy with tube in place to be sure it is endotracheal. Remove the tube immediately if there is any doubt about proper location. Secure the tube with tape and note centimeter mark at the mouth. Suction the oropharynx and trachea.
8. Confirm proper tube placement with a chest x-ray (tip of ETT should be between the carina and thoracic inlet, or level with the top of the aortic notch).

Nasotracheal Intubation

Nasotracheal intubation is the preferred method of intubation if prolonged intubation is anticipated (increased patient comfort). Intubation will be facilitated if the patient is awake and spontaneously breathing. There is an increased incidence of sinusitis with nasotracheal intubation.

1. Spray the nasal passage with a vasoconstrictor such as cocaine 4% or phenylephrine 0.25% (Neo-Synephrine). If sedation is required before nasotracheal intubation, administer midazolam (Versed) 0.05-0.1 mg/kg IV push. Lubricate the nasal airway with lidocaine ointment.
   Tube Size:
      Women 7.0 mm tube
      Men 8.0, 9.0 mm tube
2. Place the nasotracheal tube into the nasal passage, and guide it into nasopharynx along a U-shaped path. Monitor breath sounds by listening and feeling the end of tube. As the tube enters the oropharynx, gradually guide the tube downward. If the breath sounds stop, withdraw the tube 1-2 cm until breath sounds are heard again. Reposition the tube, and, if necessary, extend the head and advance. If difficulty is encountered, perform direct laryngoscopy and insert tube under direct visualization.
3. Successful intubation occurs when the tube passes through the cords; a cough may occur and breath sounds will reach maximum intensity if the tube is correctly positioned. Confirm correct placement by checking for bilateral breath sounds and expansion of the chest.
4. Confirm proper tube placement with chest x-ray.

Respiratory Failure and Ventilator Management

I. **Indications for ventilatory support**. Respirations >35, vital capacity <15 mL/kg, negative inspiratory force <-25, pO_2 <60 on 50% O_2. pH <7.2, pCO_2 >55, severe, progressive, symptomatic hypercapnia and/or hypoxia, severe metabolic acidosis.

II. **Initiation of ventilator support**
   A. **Noninvasive positive pressure ventilation** may be safely utilized in acute hypercapnic respiratory failure, avoiding the need for invasive ventilation and accompanying complications. It is not useful in normocapnic or hypoxemic respiratory failure.
   B. **Intubation**
      1. **Prepare suction apparatus**, laryngoscope, endotracheal tube (No. 8); clear airway and place oral airway, hyperventilate with bag and mask attached to high-flow oxygen.
      2. **Midazolam (Versed)** 1-2 mg IV boluses until sedated.
      3. **Intubate**, inflate cuff, ventilate with bag, auscultate chest, and suction trachea.
   C. **Initial orders**
      1. **Assist control (AC)** 8-14 breaths/min, tidal volume = 750 mL (6 cc/kg ideal body weight), FiO_2 = 100%, PEEP = 3-5 cm H_2O, Set rate so that minute ventilation (VE) is approximately 10 L/min. Alternatively, use intermittent mandatory ventilation (IMV) mode with same

tidal volume and rate to achieve near-total ventilatory support. Pressure support at 5-15 cm H_2O in addition to IMV may be added.

2. **ABG** should be obtained. Check ABG for adequate ventilation and oxygenation. If PO_2 is adequate and pulse oximetry is >98%, then titrate FiO_2 to a safe level (FIO_2<60%) by observing the saturation via pulse oximetry. Repeat ABG when target FiO_2 is reached.

3. **Chest x-ray for tube placement**, measure cuff pressure q8h (maintain <20 mm Hg), pulse oximeter, arterial line, and/or monitor end tidal CO_2. Maintain oxygen saturation >90-95%.

Ventilator Management

A. **Decreased minute ventilation.** Evaluate patient and rule out complications (endotracheal tube malposition, cuff leak, excessive secretions, bronchospasms, pneumothorax, worsening pulmonary disease, sedative drugs, pulmonary infection). Readjust ventilator rate to maintain mechanically assisted minute ventilation of 10 L/min. If peak airway pressure (AWP) is >45 cm H_2O, decrease tidal volume to 7-8 L/kg (with increase in rate if necessary), or decrease ventilator flow rate.

B. **Arterial saturation >94% and pO_2 >100**, reduce FIO_2 (each 1% decrease in FIO_2 reduces pO_2 by 7 mm Hg); once FIO_2 is <60%, PEEP may be reduced by increments of 2 cm H_2O until PEEP is 3-5cm H_2O. Maintain O_2 saturation of >90% (pO_2 >60).

C. **Arterial saturation <90% and pO_2 <60**, increase FIO_2 up to 60-100%, then consider increasing PEEP by increments of 3-5 cm H_2O (PEEP >10 requires a PA catheter). Add additional PEEP until oxygenation is adequate with an FIO_2 of <60%.

D. **Excessively low pH,** (pH <7.33 because of respiratory acidosis/hypercapnia): Increase rate and/or tidal volume. Keep peak airway pressure <40-50 cm H_2O if possible.

E. **Excessively high pH** (>7.48 because of respiratory alkalosis/hypocapnia): Reduce rate and/or tidal volume. If the patient is breathing rapidly above ventilator rate, consider sedation.

F. **Patient "fighting ventilator":** Consider IMV or SIMV mode, or add sedation with or without paralysis. Paralytic agents should not be used without concurrent amnesia and/or sedation.

G. **Sedation**
   1. **Midazolam (Versed)** 0.05 mg/kg IVP x1, then 0.02-0.1 mg/kg/hr IV infusion. Titrate in increments of 25-50%.
   2. **Lorazepam (Ativan)** 1-2 mg IV ql-2h pm sedation or 0.05 mg/kg IVP x1, then 0.025-0.2 mg/kg/hr IV infusion. Titrate in increments of 25-50%.
   3. **Morphine sulfate** 2-5 mg IV q1h or 0.03-0.05 mg/kg/h IV infusion (100 mg in 250 mL D5W) titrated.
   4. **Propofol (Diprivan):** 50 mcg/kg bolus over 5 min, then 5-50 mcg/kg/min. Titrate in increments of 5 mcg/kg/min.

H. **Paralysis** (with simultaneous amnesia)
   1. **Vecuronium (Norcuron)** 0.1 mg/kg IV, then 0.06 mg/kg/h IV infusion; intermediate acting, maximum neuromuscular blockade within 3-5 min. Half-life 60 min, **OR**

2. **Cisatracurium (Nimbex)** 0.15 mg/kg IV, then 0.3 mcg/kg/min IV infusion, titrate between 0.5-10 mcg/kg/min. Intermediate acting with half-life of 25 minutes. Drug of choice for patients with renal or liver impairment, **OR**

3. **Pancuronium (Pavulon)** 0.08 mg/kg IV, then 0.03 mg/kg/h infusion. Long acting, half-life 110 minutes; may cause tachycardia and/or hypertension, **OR**

4. **Atracurium (Tracrium)** 0.5 mg/kg IV, then 0.3-0.6 mg/kg/h infusion, short acting; half-life 20 minutes. Histamine releasing properties may cause bronchospasm and/or hypotension.

5. Monitor level of paralysis with a peripheral nerve stimulator. Adjust neuromuscular blocker dosage to achieve a "train-of-four" (TOF) of 90-95%; if inverse ratio ventilation is being used, maintain TOF at 100%.

I. **Loss at tidal volume:** If a difference between the tidal volume setting and the delivered volume occurs, check for a leak in the ventilator or inspiratory line. Check for a poor seal between the endotracheal tube cuff or malposition of the cuff in the subglottic area. If a chest tube is present, check for air leak.

J. **High peak pressure:** If peak pressure is >40-50, consider bronchospasm, secretion, pneumothorax, ARDS, agitation. Suction the patient and auscultate lungs. Obtain chest radiograph if pneumothorax, pneumonia or ARDS is suspected. Check "plateau pressure" to differentiate airway resistance from compliance causes.

Inverse Ratio Ventilation

1. Indications: ARDS physiology, pAO_2 <60 mm Hg, FIO_2 >0.6, peak airway pressure >45 cm H_2O, or PEEP > 15 cm H_2O. This type of ventilatory support requires heavy sedation and respiratory muscle relaxation.

2. Set oxygen concentration (FIO_2) at 1.0; inspiratory pressure at ½ to ⅓ of the peak airway pressure on standard ventilation. Set the inspiration: expiration ratio at 1: 1; set rate at <15 breaths/min. Maintain tidal volume by adjusting inspiratory pressures.

3. Monitor PaO_2, oxygen saturation (by pulse oximetry), $PaCO_2$, end tidal PCO_2, PEEP, mean airway pressure, heart rate, blood pressure, SVO_2, and cardiac output.

4. It SaO_2 remains <0.9, consider increasing I:E ratio (2:1, 3:1), but attempt to keep I:E ratio <2:1. If SaO_2 remains <0.9, increase PEEP or return to conventional mode. If hypotension develops, rule out tension pneumothorax, administer intravascular volume or pressor agents, decrease I:E ratio, or return to conventional ventilation mode.

Ventilator Weaning

I. **Ventilator weaning parameters**
   A. Patient alert and rested
   B. PaO_2 >70 mm Hg on FiO_2 <50%
   C. $PaCO_2$ <50 mm Hg; pH >7.25
   D. Negative Inspiratory Force (NIF) less than -40 cm H_2O
   E. Vital Capacity >10-15 mL/kg (800-1000 mL)

F. Minute Ventilation (VE) <10 L/min; respirations <24 breaths per min
G. Maximal voluntary minute (MVV) ventilation doubles that of resting minute ventilation (VE).
H. PEEP <5 cm H_2O
I. Tidal volume 5-8 mL/kg
J. Respiratory rate to tidal volume ratio <105
K. No chest wall or cardiovascular instability or excessive secretions

II. Weaning protocols

A. Weaning is considered when patient medical condition (ie, cardiac, pulmonary) status has stabilized.

B. **Indications for termination of weaning trial**
   1. PaO_2 falls below 55 mm Hg
   2. Acute hypercapnia
   3. Deterioration of vital signs or clinical status (arrhythmia)

C. **Rapid T-tube weaning method for short-term (<7 days) ventilator patients without COPD**
   1. **Obtain baseline respiratory rate, pulse, blood pressure** and arterial blood gases or oximetry. Discontinue sedation, have the well-rested patient sit in bed or chair. Provide bronchodilators and suctioning if needed.
   2. **Attach endotracheal tube** to a T-tube with FiO_2 >10% greater than previous level. Set T-tube flow-by rate to exceed peak inspiratory flow.
   3. **Patients who are tried on T-tube trial** should be observed closely for signs of deterioration. After initial 15-minute interval of spontaneous ventilation, resume mechanical ventilation and check oxygen saturation or draw an arterial blood gas sample.
   4. **If the 30-minute blood gas is acceptable,** a 60-minute interval may be attempted. After each interval, the patient is placed back on the ventilator for an equal amount of time.
   5. **If the 60-minute interval blood gas is acceptable** and the patient is without dyspnea, and if blood gases are acceptable, extubation may be considered.

D. **Pressure support ventilation weaning method**
   1. **Pressure support ventilation is initiated at 5-25 cm H_2O.** Set level to maintain the spontaneous tidal volume at 7-15 mL/kg.
   2. **Gradually decrease the level of pressure support ventilation** in increments of 3-5 cm H_2O according to the ability of the patient to maintain satisfactory minute ventilation.
   3. **Extubation** can be considered at a pressure support ventilation level of 5 cm H_2O provided that the patient can maintain stable respiratory status and blood gasses.

E. **Intermittent mandatory ventilation (IMV) weaning method**
   1. **Obtain baseline vital signs and draw baseline arterial blood gases** or pulse oximetry. Discontinue sedation; consider adding pressure support of 10-15 cm H_2O.
   2. **Change the ventilator from assist control to IMV mode**; or if already on IMV mode, decrease the rate as follows:
      a. **Patients with no underlying lung disease** and on ventilator for a brief period (<1 week).
         (1) Decrease IMV rate at 30 min intervals by 1-3 breath per min at each step, starting at rate of 8-10 until a rate for zero is reached.

       (2) If each step is tolerated and ABG is adequate (pH >7.3-7.35), extubation may be considered.

       (3) Alternatively: The patient may be watched on minimal support (ie, pressure support with CPAP) after IMV rate of zero is reached. If no deterioration is noted, extubation may be accomplished.

  b. Patients with COPD or prolonged ventilator support (>1 week)

       (1) Begin with IMV at frequency of 8 breath/minute, with tidal volume of 10 mL/kg, with an FiO_2 10% greater than previous setting. Check end-tidal CO_2.

       (2) ABG should be drawn at 30- and 60-minute intervals to check for adequate ventilation and oxygenation. If the patient and/or blood gas deteriorate during weaning trial, then return to previous stable setting.

       (3) Decrease IMV rate in increments of 1-2 breath per hour if the patient is clinical status and blood gases remain stable. Check ABG and saturation one-half hour after a new rate is set.

       (4) If the patient tolerates an IMV rate of zero, decrease the pressure to support in increments of 2-5 cm H_2O per hour until a pressure support of 5 cm H_2O is reached.

       (5) Observe the patient for an additional 24 hours on minimal support before extubation.

3. Causes of inability to wean patients from ventilators: Bronchospasm, active pulmonary infection, secretions, small endotracheal tube, weakness of respiratory muscle, low cardiac output.

Pulmonary Embolism

Approximately 300,000 Americans suffer pulmonary embolism each year. Among those in whom the condition is diagnosed, 2 percent die within the first day and 10 percent have recurrent pulmonary embolism.

I. Diagnosis of pulmonary embolism

  A. Pulmonary embolism should be suspected in any patient with new cardiopulmonary symptoms or signs and significant risk factors. If no other satisfactory explanation can be found in a patient with findings suggestive of pulmonary embolism, the workup for PE must be pursued to completion.

  B. Signs and symptoms of pulmonary embolism. Pleuritic chest pain, unexplained shortness of breath, tachycardia, hypoxemia, hypotension, hemoptysis, cough, syncope. The classic triad of dyspnea, chest pain, and hemoptysis is seen in only 20% of patients. The majority of patients have only a few subtle symptoms or are asymptomatic.

  C. Massive pulmonary emboli may cause the sudden onset of precordial pain, dyspnea, syncope, or shock. Other findings include distended neck veins, cyanosis, diaphoresis, pre-cordial heave, a loud pulmonic valve component of the second heart sound. Right ventricular S3, and a tricuspid insufficiency.

  D. Deep venous thrombosis may manifest as an edematous limb with an erythrocyanotic appearance, dilated superficial veins, and elevated skin temperature.

Frequency of Symptoms and Signs in Pulmonary Embolism			
Symptoms	**Frequency (%)**	**Signs**	**Frequency (%)**
Dyspnea	84	Tachypnea (>16/min)	92
Pleuritic chest pain	74	Rales	58
Apprehension	59	Accentuated S2	53
Cough	53	Tachycardia	44
Hemoptysis	30	Fever (>37.8°C)	43
Sweating	27	Diaphoresis	36
Non-pleuritic chest pain	14	S3 or S4 gallop	34
		Thrombophlebitis	32

II. **Risk factors for pulmonary embolism**
   A. **Venous stasis.** Prolonged immobilization, hip surgery, stroke, myocardial infarction, heart failure, obesity, varicose veins, anesthesia, age >65 years old.
   B. **Endothelial injury.** Surgery, trauma, central venous access catheters, pacemaker wires, previous thromboembolic event.
   C. **Hypercoagulable state.** Malignant disease, high estrogen level (oral contraceptives).
   D. **Hematologic disorders.** Polycythemia, leukocytosis, thrombocytosis, antithrombin III deficiency, protein C deficiency, protein S deficiency, antiphospholipid syndrome, inflammatory bowel disease, factor 5 Leiden defect.

III. **Diagnostic evaluation**
   A. **Chest radiographs** are nonspecific and insensitive, and findings are normal in up to 40 percent of patients with pulmonary embolism. Abnormalities may include an elevated hemidiaphragm, focal infiltrates, atelectasis, and small pleural effusions.
   B. **Electrocardiography** is nonspecific and often normal. The most common abnormality is sinus tachycardia. Other findings may include ST-segment or T-wave changes. Occasionally, acute right ventricular strain causes tall peaked P waves in lead II, right axis deviation, right bundle branch block, or atrial fibrillation.
   C. **Blood gas studies.** There is no level of arterial oxygen that can rule out pulmonary embolism. Most patients with pulmonary embolism have a normal arterial oxygen.
   D. **Ventilation-perfusion scan**
      1. Patients with a clearly normal perfusion scan do not have a pulmonary embolism, and less than 5 percent of patients with near-normal scan have a pulmonary embolism. A high-probability scan has a 90 percent probability of a pulmonary embolism.
      2. **A low-probability V/Q scan** can exclude the diagnosis of pulmonary embolism only if the patient has a clinically low probability of pulmonary embolism.
      3. **Intermediate V/Q scans** are not diagnostic and usually indicate the need for further diagnostic testing. One-third of patients with intermediate scans have a pulmonary embolism and should have a follow-up chest CT or pulmonary angiography.

E. Venous imaging

1. If the V/Q scan is nondiagnostic, a workup for deep venous thrombosis (DVT) should be pursued using duplex ultrasound. The identification of DVT in a patient with signs and symptoms suggesting pulmonary embolism proves the diagnosis of pulmonary embolism. A deep venous thrombosis can be found in 80% of cases of pulmonary emboli.

2. Inability to demonstrate the existence of a DVT does not significantly lower the likelihood of pulmonary embolism because clinically asymptomatic DVT may not be detectable.

3. Patients with a nondiagnostic V/Q scan and no demonstrable site of DVT should proceed to chest CT or pulmonary angiography.

F. Chest CT may be used in place of pulmonary angiography in patients with abnormal chest x-ray in whom V/Q scan is nondiagnostic, or in presence of an intermediate probability of PE on V/Q scan. Chest CT is associated with fewer complications than pulmonary angiography. However, chest CT offers a more limited view of this pulmonary field and does not allow for measurement of pulmonary artery pressure.

G. Angiography. Contrast pulmonary arteriography is the "gold standard" for the diagnosis of pulmonary embolism. False-negative results occur in 2-10% of patients. Angiography carries a low risk of complications (minor 5%, major nonfatal 1%, fatal 0.5%).

IV. Management of acute pulmonary embolism in stable patients

A. Oxygen should be initiated for all patients.

B. Antithrombotic therapy

1. Heparin therapy should be started as soon as the diagnosis of pulmonary embolism is suspected. Full-dose heparin can be given immediately after major surgery.

2. **Unfractionated heparin** is administrated as 80 U/kg IVP, then 18 U/kg/h IV infusion. Obtain an aPTT in 6 hours, and adjust dosage based on the table below to maintain the aPTT between 60-85 seconds. Contraindications to heparin include active internal bleeding and recent and significant trauma.

Heparin Maintenance Dose Adjustment				
aPTTs	Bolus Dose	Stop infusion	Rate Change, mL/h*	Repeat aPTT
<50	5000 U	0 min	+3 (increase by 150 U/h)	6 h
50-59	0	0 min	+2 (increase by 100 U/h)	6 h
60-85	0	0 min	0 (no change)	next AM
86-95	0	0 min	-1 (decrease by 50 U/h)	next AM
96-120	0	30 min	-2 (decrease by 100 U/h)	6 h

aPTTs	Bolus Dose	Stop infusion	Rate Change, mL/h*	Repeat aPTT
>120	0	60 min	-3 (decrease by 150 U/h)	6 h
*50 U/mL				

3. Platelet count should be monitored during heparin therapy; thrombocytopenia develops in 5% of patients after 3-7 days of therapy. Heparin may rarely induce hyperkalemia, which resolves spontaneously upon discontinuation.

4. **Low-molecular-weight heparin (LMWH)** is as effective as unfractionated heparin for uncomplicated PE. It does not require monitoring and may allow for earlier hospital discharge. Enoxaparin (Lovenox) can be used for DVT with uncomplicated PE: 1 mg/kg SC q12h x 5 day minimum. Therapy with LMWH should overlap warfarin for 3-4 days.

5. **Warfarin (Coumadin)** may be started as soon as the diagnosis of pulmonary embolism is confirmed and heparin has been initiated. Starting dose is 10 mg PO qd for 3 days. The dose is then adjusted to keep the International Normalized Ratio (INR) at 2.0-3.0. The typical dosage is 2.0-7.5 mg PO qd. Heparin and warfarin regimens are overlapped for 3 to 5 days until the INR is 2.0-3.0, then heparin is discontinued.

6. Therapy with warfarin is generally continued for 3-6 months. In patients with an ongoing risk factor or following a second episode of DVT, life-long anticoagulation with warfarin may be necessary.

C. **Thrombolysis**

1. Unstable patients (systolic <90 mm Hg) with proven pulmonary embolism require immediate clot lysis by thrombolytic therapy. Tissue plasminogen activator (Activase) is recommended because it is the fastest-acting thrombolytic agent.

2. **Contraindications to thrombolytics**
   a. **Absolute contraindications.** Active bleeding, cerebrovascular accident or surgery within the past 2 months, intracranial neoplasms.
   b. **Relative contraindications.** Recent gastrointestinal bleeding, uncontrolled hypertension, recent trauma (cardiopulmonary resuscitation), pregnancy.

3. **Alteplase (tPA, Activase).** 100 mg by peripheral IV infusion over 2 hr. Heparin therapy should be initiated after cessation of the thrombolytic infusion. Heparin is started without a loading dose at 18 U/kg/hr when the aPTT is 1.5 times control rate.

D. **Fluid and pharmacologic management.** In acute cor pulmonale, gentle pharmacologic preload reduction with furosemide unloads the congested pulmonary circuit and reduces right ventricular pressures. Hydralazine, isoproterenol, or norepinephrine may be required. Pulmonary artery pressure monitoring may be helpful.

E. **Emergency thoracotomy.** Emergency surgical removal of embolized thrombus is reserved for instances when there is an absolute contraindication to thrombolysis or when the patient's condition has failed to improve after thrombolysis. Cardiac arrest from pulmonary embolism is an indication for immediate thoracotomy.

Asthma

Asthma is the most common chronic disease among children. Asthma triggers include viral infections; environmental pollutants, such as tobacco smoke; aspirin, nonsteroidal anti-inflammatory drugs, and sustained exercise, particularly in cold environments.

I. **Diagnosis**
  A. Symptoms of asthma may include episodic complaints of breathing difficulties, seasonal or nighttime cough, prolonged shortness of breath after a respiratory infection, or difficulty sustaining exercise.
  B. Wheezing does not always represent asthma. Wheezing may persist for weeks after an acute bronchitis episode. Patients with chronic obstructive pulmonary disease may have a reversible component superimposed on their fixed obstruction. Etiologic clues include a personal history of allergic disease, such as rhinitis or atopic dermatitis, and a family history of allergic disease.
  C. The frequency of daytime and nighttime symptoms, duration of exacerbations and asthma triggers should be assessed.
  D. **Physical examination.** Hyperventilation, use of accessory muscles of respiration, audible wheezing, and a prolonged expiratory phase are common. Increased nasal secretions or congestion, polyps, and eczema may be present.
  E. **Measurement of lung function.** An increase in the forced expiratory volume in one second (FEV_1) of 12% after treatment with an inhaled beta$_2$ agonist is sufficient to make the diagnosis of asthma. A 12% change in peak expiratory flow rate (PEFR) measured on a peak-flow meter is also diagnostic.

II. **Treatment of asthma**
  A. **Beta$_2$ agonists**
    1. Inhaled short-acting beta$_2$-adrenergic agonists are the most effective drugs available for treatment of acute bronchospasm and for prevention of exercise-induced asthma. Levalbuterol, the R-isomer of racemic albuterol, offers no significant advantage over racemic albuterol.
    2. Salmeterol, a long-acting beta$_2$ agonist, has a relatively slow onset of action and a prolonged effect. Salmeterol should not be used in the treatment of acute bronchospasm. Patients taking salmeterol should use a short-acting beta$_2$ agonist as needed to control acute symptoms. Twice-daily inhalation of salmeterol has been effective for maintenance treatment in combination with inhaled corticosteroids.
    3. **Adverse effects of beta$_2$ agonists.** Tachycardia, palpitations, tremor and paradoxical bronchospasm can occur. High doses can cause hypokalemia.

Drugs for Asthma

Drug	Formulation	Dosage
Inhaled beta$_2$-adrenergic agonists, short-acting		
Albuterol *Proventil* *Proventil-HFA* *Ventolin* *Ventolin Rotacaps*	metered-dose inhaler (90 μg/puff) dry-powder inhaler (200 μg/inhalation)	2 puffs q4-6h PRN 1-2 capsules q4-6h PRN
Albuterol *Proventil* multi-dose vials *Ventolin Nebules* *Ventolin*	nebulized	2.5 mg q4-6h PRN
Levalbuterol - *Xopenex*	nebulized	0.63-1.25 mg q6-8h PRN
Inhaled beta2-adrenergic agonist, long-acting		
Salmeterol *Serevent* *Serevent Diskus*	metered-dose inhaler (21 μg/puff) dry-powder inhaler (50 μg/inhalation)	2 puffs q12h 1 inhalation q12h
Inhaled Corticosteroids		
Beclomethasone dipropionate *Beclovent* *Vanceril* Vanceril Double-Strength	metered-dose inhaler (42 μg/puff) (84 μg/puff)	4-8 puffs bid 2-4 puffs bid
Budesonide *Pulmicort Turbuhaler*	dry-powder inhaler (200 μg/inhalation)	1-2 inhalations bid
Flunisolide - *AeroBid*	metered-dose inhaler (250 μg/puff)	2-4 puffs bid
Fluticasone Flovent *Flovent Rotadisk*	metered-dose inhaler (44, 110 or 220 μg/puff) dry-powder inhaler (50, 100 or 250 μg/inhalation)	2-4 puffs bid (44 μg/puff) 1 inhalation bid (100 μg/inhalation)
Triamcinolone acetonide *Azmacort*	metered-dose inhaler (100 μg/puff)	2 puffs tid-qid or 4 puffs bid
Leukotriene Modifiers		
Montelukast - *Singulair*	tablets	10 mg qhs

Drug	Formulation	Dosage
Zafirlukast - *Accolate*	tablets	20 mg bid
Zileuton - *Zyflo*	tablets	600 mg qid
Mast Cell Stabilizers		
Cromolyn *Intal*	metered-dose inhaler (800 µg/puff)	2-4 puffs tid-qid
Nedocromil *Tilade*	metered-dose inhaler (1.75 mg/puff)	2-4 puffs bid-qid
Phosphodiesterase Inhibitor		
Theophylline *Slo-Bid Gyrocaps, Theo-Dur, Unidur*	extended-release capsules or tablets	100-300 mg bid

B. Inhaled corticosteroids
 1. Regular use of an inhaled corticosteroid can suppress inflammation, decrease bronchial hyperresponsiveness and decrease symptoms. Inhaled corticosteroids are recommended for treatment of patients with mild or moderate persistent asthma as well as those with severe disease.
 2. **Adverse effects.** Inhaled corticosteroids are usually free of toxicity. Dose-dependent slowing of linear growth may occur within 6-12 weeks in some children. Decreased bone density, glaucoma and cataract formation have been reported. Churg-Strauss vasculitis has been reported rarely. Dysphonia and oral candidiasis can occur. The use of a spacer device and rinsing the mouth after inhalation decreases the incidence of candidiasis.

C. Leukotriene modifiers
 1. Leukotrienes increase production of mucus and edema of the airway wall, and may cause bronchoconstriction. Montelukast and zafirlukast are leukotriene receptor antagonists. Zileuton inhibits synthesis of leukotrienes.
 2. **Montelukast (Singulair)** is modestly effective for maintenance treatment of intermittent or persistent asthma. It is taken once daily in the evening. It is less effective than inhaled corticosteroids, but addition of montelukast may permit a reduction in corticosteroid dosage. Montelukast added to oral or inhaled corticosteroids can improve symptoms.
 3. **Zafirlukast (Accolate)** is modestly effective for maintenance treatment of mild-to-moderate asthma It is less effective than inhaled corticosteroids. Taking zafirlukast with food markedly decreases its bioavailability. Theophylline can decrease its effect. Zafirlukast increases serum concentrations of oral anticoagulants and may cause bleeding. Infrequent adverse effects include mild headache, gastrointestinal disturbances and increased serum aminotransferase activity. Drug-induced lupus and Churg-Strauss vasculitis have been reported.

    4. Zileuton (Zyflo) is modestly effective for maintenance treatment, but it is taken four times a day and patients must be monitored for hepatic toxicity.

D. Cromolyn (Intal) and nedocromil (Tilade)

    1. Cromolyn sodium, an inhibitor of mast cell degranulation, can decrease airway hyperresponsiveness in some patients with asthma. The drug has no bronchodilating activity and is useful only for prophylaxis. Cromolyn has virtually no systemic toxicity.

    2. Nedocromil has similar effects as cromolyn. Both cromolyn and nedocromil are much less effective than inhaled corticosteroids.

E. Theophylline

    1. Oral theophylline has a slower onset of action than inhaled beta$_2$ agonists and has limited usefulness for treatment of acute symptoms. It can, however, reduce the frequency and severity of symptoms, especially in nocturnal asthma, and can decrease inhaled corticosteroid requirements.

    2. When theophylline is used alone, serum concentrations between 8-12 mcg/mL provide a modest improvement is FEV$_1$. Serum levels of 15-20 mcg/mL are only minimally more effective and are associated with a higher incidence of cardiovascular adverse events.

F. Oral corticosteroids are the most effective drugs available for acute exacerbations of asthma unresponsive to bronchodilators.

    1. Oral corticosteroids decrease symptoms and may prevent an early relapse. Chronic use of oral corticosteroids can cause glucose intolerance, weight gain, increased blood pressure, osteoporosis, cataracts, immunosuppression and decreased growth in children. Alternate-day use of corticosteroids can decrease the incidence of adverse effects, but not of osteoporosis.

    2. Prednisone, prednisolone or methylprednisolone (Solu-Medrol), 40-60 mg qd; for children, 1-2 mg/kg/day to a maximum of 60 mg/day. Therapy is continued for 3-10 days. The oral steroid dosage does not need to be tapered after short-course "burst" therapy if the patient is receiving inhaled steroid therapy.

G. Choice of drugs

    1. Patients with infrequent mild symptoms of asthma may require only intermittent use, as needed, of a short-acting inhaled beta$_2$-adrenergic agonist. Overuse of inhaled short-acting beta$_2$ agonists or more than twice a week indicates that an inhaled corticosteroid should be added to the treatment regimen.

Pharmacotherapy for Asthma Based on Disease Classification		
Classification	Long-term control medications	Quick-relief medications
Mild intermittent		Short-acting beta$_2$ agonist as needed
Mild persistent	Low-dose inhaled corticosteroid or cromolyn sodium (Intal) or nedocromil (Tilade)	Short-acting beta$_2$ agonist as needed

Classification	Long-term control medications	Quick-relief medications
Moderate persistent	Medium-dose inhaled corticosteroid plus a long-acting bronchodilator (long-acting beta$_2$ agonist)	Short-acting beta$_2$ agonist as needed
Severe persistent	High-dose inhaled corticosteroid plus a long-acting bronchodilator and systemic corticosteroid	Short-acting beta$_2$ agonist as needed

III. Management of acute exacerbations

- **A.** High-dose, short-acting beta$_2$ agonists delivered by a metered-dose inhaler with a volume spacer or via a nebulizer remains the mainstay of urgent treatment.
- **B.** Most patients require therapy with systemic corticosteroids to resolve symptoms and prevent relapse.
- **C.** Hospitalization should be considered if the PEFR remains less than 70% of predicted. Patients with a PEFR less than 50% of predicted who exhibit an increasing pCO$_2$ level and declining mental status are candidates for intubation.
- **D.** Non-invasive ventilation with bilevel positive airway pressure (BIPAP) may be used to relieve the work-of-breathing while awaiting the effects of acute treatment, provided that consciousness and the ability to protect the airway have not been compromised.

Chronic Obstructive Pulmonary Disease

Chronic obstructive pulmonary disease affects more than 20 million Americans. This condition is composed of three distinct entities: 1) chronic bronchitis; 2) emphysema; and 3) peripheral airway disease. The greatest percentage of patients with COPD have chronic bronchitis.

I. Clinical evaluation

- **A.** The majority of patients with COPD will have either a history of cigarette smoking or exposure to second-hand cigarette smoke. Occasionally, patients will develop COPD from occupational exposure. A minority of patients develop emphysema as a result of alpha-1-protease inhibitor deficiency or intravenous drug abuse.
- **B.** The patient with acute exacerbations of COPD (AECOPD) usually will complain of cough, sputum production, and/or dyspnea. Acute exacerbations may be precipitated by an infectious process, exposure to noxious stimuli, or environmental changes. It is important to compare the current illness with the severity of previous episodes and to determine if the patient has had previous intubations or admissions to the ICU.
- **C.** Intercostal retractions, accessory muscle use, and an increase in pulsus paradoxus usually suggest significant airway obstruction.
- **D.** Wheezing is usually present. Emphysema is manifested by an elongated, hyperresonant chest. Diaphragmatic flattening and increased radiolucency is seen on the chest x-ray.

II. Infectious precipitants of acute exacerbations of COPD

A. About 32% of patients with an acute exacerbation have a viral infection. The most common agents are influenza virus, parainfluenzae, and respiratory syncytial virus.

B. Bacterial precipitants play an important etiologic role in AECOPD. H. influenzae is the most common pathogen, occurring in 19%, followed by Streptococcus pneumoniae in 12% and Moraxella catarrhalis in 8%. Patients with COPD have chronic colonization of the respiratory tree with Streptococcus pneumoniae, Haemophilus influenzae, and Haemophilus parainfluenzae.

III. Diagnostic testing

A. **Pulse oximetry** is an inexpensive, noninvasive procedure for assessing oxygen saturation.

B. **Arterial blood gases.** Both hypercarbia and hypoxemia occur when pulmonary function falls to below 25-30% of the predicted normal value.

C. **Pulmonary function testing** is a useful means for assessing ventilatory function. Peak-flow meters are available that can provide a quick assessment of expiratory function.

D. **Chest radiography** will permit identification of patients with COPD with pneumonia, pneumothorax, and decompensated CHF.

E. **An ECG** may be useful in patients who have a history of chest pain, syncope, and palpitations.

F. **Labs:** Complete blood count (CBC) is useful in patients with acute exacerbation of COPD if pneumonia is suspected. The hematocrit is frequently elevated as a result of chronic hypoxemia. A serum theophylline level should be obtained in patients who are taking theophylline. Each milligram per kilogram of theophylline raises the serum theophylline level by about 2 mcg/mL.

IV. Pharmacotherapy for patient stabilization

A. **Oxygen.** Patients in respiratory distress should receive supplemental oxygen therapy. Oxygen therapy usually is initiated by nasal cannula to maintain an O_2 saturation greater than 90%. Patients with hypercarbia may require controlled oxygen therapy using a Venturi mask in order to achieve more precise control of the FiO_2.

B. **Beta-agonists** are first-line therapy for AECOPD. Albuterol is the most widely used agent.

Beta-Agonist Dosages		
Agent	**MDI**	**Aerosol**
Albuterol (Proventil, Ventolin)	2-4 puffs q4h	0.5 cc (2.5 mg)
Pirbuterol (Maxair)	2 puffs q4-6h	
Salmeterol (Serevent)	2 puffs q12h	

C. **Anticholinergic agents** produce preferential dilatation of the larger central airways, in contrast to beta-agonists, which affect the peripheral airways. Ipratropium is a first-line therapeutic option for chronic, outpatient management of stable patients with COPD. The usual dose is 2-4 puffs every six hours. The inhalation dose is 500 mcg/2.5 mL solution nebulized 3-4 times daily.

D. Corticosteroids. Rapidly tapering courses of corticosteroids are effective in preventing relapses and maintaining longer symptom-free intervals in patients who have had AECOPD. Patients with an acute exacerbation of COPD should receive steroids as a mainstay of outpatient therapy. There is no role for inhaled corticosteroids in the treatment of acute exacerbations.

   1. Oral steroids are warranted in severe COPD. Prednisone 0.5-1.0 mg/kg or 40 mg qAM. The dose should be tapered over 1-2 weeks following clinical improvement.

   2. Aerosolized corticosteroids provide the benefits of oral corticosteroids with fewer side effects.
   Triamcinolone (Azmacort) MDI 2-4 puffs bid.
   Flunisolide (AeroBid, AeroBid-M) MDI 2-4 puffs bid.
   Beclomethasone (Beclovent) MDI 2-4 puffs bid.
   Budesonide (Pulmicort) MDI 2 puffs bid.

   3. **Side effects of corticosteroids.** Cataracts, osteoporosis, sodium and water retention, hypokalemia, muscle weakness, aseptic necrosis of femoral and humeral heads, peptic ulcer disease, pancreatitis, endocrine and skin abnormalities, muscle wasting.

E. Theophylline has a relatively narrow therapeutic index with side effects that range from nausea, vomiting, and tremor to more serious side effects, including seizures and ventricular arrhythmias. Dosage of long-acting theophylline (Slo-bid, Theo-Dur) is 200-300 mg bid. Theophylline preparations with 24-hour action may be administered once a day in the early evening. Theo-24, 100-400 mg qd [100, 200, 300, 400 mg].

F. Salmeterol (Serevent) is a long-acting beta-agonist, which may improve nocturnal dyspnea and reduce the frequency of beta-agonist rescue use. 2 puffs q12h.

G. Summary of therapeutic approaches
   1. **Acute exacerbations** are treated with systemic steroids, antibiotics, and inhaled beta-agonists with combined ipratropium. Lack of improvement should prompt addition of theophylline, salmeterol, non-invasive ventilatory support (BIPAP), or intubation with mechanical ventilatory support.

   2. **Chronic and stable COPD** is treated with scheduled doses of ipratropium in combination with albuterol. Salmeterol and theophylline are added when symptom control is difficult. Addition of an inhaled steroid may be beneficial in selected patients. Continuous oxygen therapy has clear benefits when indicated by a resting, exercise, or sleeping PaO_2 <55 mm Hg.

H. Antibiotics. Amoxicillin-resistant, beta-lactamase-producing H. influenzae are common. Azithromycin has an appropriate spectrum of coverage. Levofloxacin is advantageous when gram-negative bacteria or atypical organisms predominate. Amoxicillin-clavulanate has in vitro activity against beta-lactamase-producing H. influenzae and M. catarrhalis.

> **Recommended Dosing and Duration of Antibiotic Therapy for Acute Exacerbations of COPD**
>
> **Mild-to-moderate acute exacerbations of COPD**
> - Azithromycin (Zithromax): 500 mg on 1st day, 250 mg qd × 4 days or clarithromycin (Biaxin) 500 mg PO bid.
> - Amoxicillin/clavulanate (Augmentin): 500 mg tid × 10 days or 875 mg bid × 10 days.
>
> **Severe acute exacerbations of COPD**
> - Levofloxacin (Levaquin): 500 mg qd × 7-14 days
>
> **Alternative agents for treatment of uncomplicated, acute exacerbations of chronic bronchitis**
>
> - Trimethoprim/sulfamethoxazole (Bactrim, Septra): 1 DS tab PO bid 7-14 days
> - Amoxicillin (Amoxil, Wymox): 500 mg tid × 7-14 days
> - Doxycycline (Vibramycin): 100 mg bid × 7-14 days

V. **Ventilatory assistance**
   A. Patients with extreme dyspnea, discordant breathing, fatigue, inability to speak, or deteriorating mental status in the face of adequate therapy may require ventilatory assistance. Hypoxemia that does not respond to oxygen therapy or worsening of acid-base status in spite of controlled oxygen therapy may also require ventilatory assistance.
   B. **Noninvasive, nasal, or bilevel positive airway pressure (BiPAP)** may improve respiratory rate, tidal volume, and minute ventilation. Patients successfully treated with noninvasive ventilation have a lower incidence of pneumonia and sinusitis.
VI. **Surgical treatment.** Lung volume reduction surgery (LVRS) consists of surgical removal of an emphysematous bulla. This procedure can ameliorate symptoms and improve pulmonary function. Lung transplantation is reserved for those patients deemed unsuitable or too ill for LVRS.
VII. **Hypoxemia** adversely affects function and increases risk the of death, and oxygen therapy is the only treatment documented to improve survival in patients with COPD. Oxygen is usually delivered by nasal cannula at a flow rate sufficient to maintain an optimal oxygen saturation level.

Pleural Effusion

Pre-thoracentesis chest x-ray: A bilateral decubitus x-ray should be obtained before the thoracentesis. Thoracentesis is safe when fluid freely layers out and is greater than 10 mm in depth on the decubitus film.
Labs: CBC, ABG, SMA 12, protein, albumin, amylase, rheumatoid factor, ANA, ESR. INR/PTT, UA. Chest x-ray PA & LAT repeat after thoracentesis, bilateral decubitus, ECG.
Pleural fluid analysis:
   Tube 1. LDH, protein, amylase, triglyceride, glucose (10 mL).
   Tube 2. Gram stain, C&S, AFB, fungal C&S, (20-60 mL, heparinized).

Tube 3. Cell count and differential (5-10 mL, EDTA).
Tube 4. Antigen tests for S. pneumoniae, H. influenza (25-50 mL, heparinized).
Syringe. pH (2 mL collected anaerobically, heparinized on ice)
Bottle. Cytology.

Differential Diagnosis		
Pleural Fluid Parameters	**Transudate**	**Exudate**
LDH (IU)	<200	>200
Pleural LDH/serum LDH	<0.6	>0.6
Total protein (g/dL)	<3.0	>3.0
Pleural Protein/serum Protein	<0.5	>0.5

Differential Diagnosis of Transudates: Congestive heart failure, cirrhosis.
Differential Diagnosis of Exudates: Empyema, viral pleuritis, tuberculosis, neoplasm, uremia, drug reaction, asbestosis, sarcoidosis, collagen disease (lupus, rheumatoid disease), pancreatitis, subphrenic abscess.
Chylous Effusions: Triglyceride >110
Malignant Effusions: Cytology positive in 60% of effusions.
Treatment: Chest tube drainage is indicated for complicated parapneumonic effusions (pH <7.10, glucose <40 mEq/dL, LDH >1000 IU/L) and frank empyema. Rapid removal may rarely cause re-expansion pulmonary edema.

References

Ferretti GR, et al. Acute pulmonary embolism; Role of helical CT in 164 patients with intermediate probability at ventilation-perfusion scintigraphy and normal results at duplex US of the legs. Radiology 1997, 205: 453-458.

Kollef et al. The Acute Respiratory Distress syndrome. NEJM 1995,332(1):27-37

Amato et al. Effect of a protective-ventilation strategy on mortality in the ARDS. NEJM 1998,338(6)347-54

McIntyre NR. Clinically available new strategies for mechanical ventilatory support. Chest, 1993, 104(2):500-5.

Tobin MJ. Mechanical Ventilation. NEJM, 1994, 330(15): 1056-61

Esteban A et al. A Comparison of four methods of weaning patients from mechanical ventilation. NEJM, 1995, 332 (6):345-350.

The Columbus Investigators. Low-Molecular Weight Heparin in the Treatment of patients with venous thromboembolism. NEJM 1997, 337(10):657-662.

Trauma

Blanding U. Jones, MD

Pneumothorax

I. **Management of pneumothorax**
   A. **Small primary spontaneous pneumothorax (<10-15%): (not associated with underlying pulmonary diseases). If the patient is not dyspneic.**
      1. Observe for 4-8 hours and repeat a chest x-ray.
      2. If the pneumothorax does not increase in size and the patient remains asymptomatic, consider discharge home with instructions to rest and curtail all strenuous activities. The patient should return if there is an increase in dyspnea or recurrence of chest pain.
   B. **Secondary spontaneous pneumothorax (associated with underlying pulmonary pathology, emphysema) or primary spontaneous pneumothorax >15%, or if patient is symptomatic.**
      1. Give high-flow oxygen by nasal cannula. A needle thoracotomy should be placed at the anterior, second intercostal space in the midclavicular line.
      2. Anesthetize and prep the area, then insert a 16-gauge needle with an internal catheter and a 60 mL syringe, attached via a 3-way stopcock. Aspirate until no more air is aspirated. If no additional air can be aspirated, and the volume of aspirated air is <4 liters, occlude the catheter and observe for 4 hours.
      3. If symptoms abate and chest-x-ray does not show recurrence of the pneumothorax, the catheter can be removed, and the patient can be discharged home with instructions.
      4. If the aspirated air is >4 liters and additional air is aspirated without resistance, this represents an active bronchopleural fistula with continued air leak. Admission is required for insertion of a chest tube.
   C. **Traumatic pneumothorax associated with a penetrating injury, hemothorax, mechanical ventilation, tension pneumothorax, or if pneumothorax does not resolve after needle aspiration:** Give high-flow oxygen and insert a chest tube. Do not delay the management of a tension pneumothorax until radiographic confirmation; insert needle thoracotomy or chest tube immediately.
   D. **Iatrogenic pneumothorax**
      1. Iatrogenic pneumothoraces include lung puncture caused by thoracentesis or central line placement.
      2. Administer oxygen by nasal cannula.
      3. **If the pneumothorax is less than 10% and the patient is asymptomatic,** observe and repeat chest x-ray in 4 hours. If unchanged, manage expectantly with close follow-up, and repeat chest x-ray in 24 hours.
      4. **If the pneumothorax is more than 10% and/or the patient is symptomatic,** perform a tube thoracostomy under negative pressure.

II. Technique of chest tube insertion

A. Place patient in supine position, with involved side elevated 20 degrees. Abduct the arm to 90 degrees. The usual site is the fourth or fifth intercostal space, between the mid-axillary and anterior axillary line (drainage of air or free fluid). The point at which the anterior axillary fold meets the chest wall is a useful guide. Alternatively, the second or third intercostal space, in the midclavicular line, may be used for pneumothorax drainage alone (air only).

B. Cleanse the skin with Betadine iodine solution, and drape the field. Determine the intrathoracic tube distance (lateral chest wall to the apices), and mark the length of tube with a clamp.

C. Infiltrate 1% lidocaine into the skin, subcutaneous tissues, intercostal muscles, periosteum, and pleura using a 25-gauge needle. Use a scalpel to make a transverse skin incision, 2 centimeters wide, located over the rib, just inferior to the interspace where the tube will penetrate the chest wall.

D. Use a Kelly clamp to bluntly dissect a subcutaneous tunnel from the skin incision, extending just over the superior margin of the lower rib. Avoid the nerve, artery and vein located at the upper margin of the intercostal space.

E. Penetrate the pleura with the clamp, and open the pleura 1 centimeter. With a gloved finger, explore the subcutaneous tunnel, and palpate the lung medially. Exclude possible abdominal penetration, and ensure correct location within pleural space; use finger to remove any local pleural adhesions.

F. Use the Kelly clamp to grasp the tip of the thoracostomy tube (36 F, internal diameter 12 mm), and direct it into the pleural space in a posterior, superior direction for pneumothorax evacuation. Direct the tube inferiorly for pleural fluid removal. Guide the tube into the pleural space until the last hole is inside the pleural space and not inside the subcutaneous tissue.

G. Attach the tube to a underwater seal apparatus containing sterile normal saline, and adjust to 20 cm H_2O of negative pressure, or attach to suction if leak is severe. Suture the tube to the skin of the chest wall using O silk. Apply Vaseline gauze, 4 x 4 gauze sponges, and elastic tape. Obtain a chest x-ray to verify correct placement and evaluate reexpansion of the lung.

Tension Pneumothorax

I. Clinical evaluation

A. **Clinical signs:** Severe hemodynamic and/or respiratory compromise; contralaterally deviated trachea; decreased or absent breath sounds and hyperresonance to percussion on the affected side; jugular venous distention, asymmetrical chest wall motion with respiration.

B. **Radiologic signs:** Flattening or inversion of the ipsilateral hemidiaphragm; contralateral shifting of the mediastinum; flattening of the cardio-mediastinal contour and spreading of the ribs on the ipsilateral side.

II. Acute management

A. A temporary large-bore IV catheter may be inserted into the ipsilateral pleural space, at the level of the second intercostal space at the midclavicular line until the chest tube is placed.

B. A chest tube should be placed emergently.

C. Draw blood for CBC, INR, PTT, type and cross-matching, chem 7, toxicology screen.

D. Send pleural fluid for hematocrit, amylase and pH (to rule out esophageal rupture).

E. **Indications for cardiothoracic exploration:** Severe or persistent hemodynamic instability despite aggressive fluid resuscitation, persistent active blood loss from chest tube, more than 200 cc/hr for 3 consecutive hours, or ≥ 1½ L of acute blood loss after chest tube placement.

Cardiac Tamponade

I. General considerations

A. Cardiac tamponade occurs most commonly secondary to penetrating injuries.

B. **Beck's Triad:** Venous pressure elevation, drop in the arterial pressure, muffled heart sounds. Other signs include enlarged cardiac silhouette on chest x-ray; signs and symptoms of hypovolemic shock; pulseless electrical activity, decreased voltage on ECG.

C. Kussmaul's sign is characterized by a rise in venous pressure with inspiration. Pulsus paradoxus or elevated venous pressure may be absent when associated with hypovolemia.

II. Management

A. Pericardiocentesis is indicated if the patient is unresponsive to resuscitation measures for hypovolemic shock, or if there is a high likelihood of injury to the myocardium or one of the great vessels.

B. All patients who have a positive pericardiocentesis (recovery of non-clotting blood) because of trauma, require an open thoracotomy with inspection of the myocardium and the great vessels.

C. Rule out other causes of cardiac tamponade such as pericarditis, penetration of central line through the vena cava, atrium, or ventricle, or infection.

D. Consider other causes of hemodynamic instability that may mimic cardiac tamponade (tension pneumothorax, massive pulmonary embolism, shock secondary to massive hemothorax).

Pericardiocentesis

I. General considerations

A. If acute cardiac tamponade with hemodynamic instability is suspected, emergency pericardiocentesis should be performed; infusion of Ringer's lactate, crystalloid, colloid and/or blood may provide temporizing measures.

II. Management

   A. Protect airway and administer oxygen. If patient can be stabilized, pericardiocentesis should be performed in the operating room or catheter lab. The para-xiphoid approach is used for pericardiocentesis.

   B. Place patient in supine position with chest elevated at 30-45 degrees, then cleanse and drape peri-xiphoid area. Infiltrate lidocaine 1% with epinephrine (if time permits) into skin and deep tissues.

   C. Attach a long, large bore (12-18 cm, 16-18 gauge), short bevel cardiac needle to a 50 cc syringe with a 3-way stop cock. Use an alligator clip to attach a V-lead of the ECG to the metal of the needle.

   D. Advance the needle just below costal margin, immediately to the left and inferior to the xiphoid process. Apply suction to the syringe while advancing the needle slowly at a 45 -degree horizontal angle towards the mid point of the left clavicle.

   E. As the needle penetrates the pericardium, resistance will be felt, and a "popping" sensation will be noted.

   F. Monitor the ECG for ST segment elevation (indicating ventricular heart muscle contact); or PR segment elevation (indicating atrial epicardial contact). After the needle comes in contact with the epicardium, withdraw the needle slightly. Ectopic ventricular beats are associated with cardiac penetration.

   G. Aspirate as much blood as possible. Blood from the pericardial space usually will not clot. Blood, inadvertently, drawn from inside the ventricles or atrium usually will clot. If fluid is not obtained, redirect the needle more towards the head. Stabilize the needle by attaching a hemostat or Kelly clamp.

   H. Consider emergency thoracotomy to determine the cause of hemopericardium (especially if active bleeding). If the patient does not improve, consider other problems that may resemble tamponade, such as tension pneumothorax, pulmonary embolism, or shock secondary to massive hemothorax.

References

Committee on Trauma, American College of Surgeons: Early Care of the Injured Patient. Philadelphia, WB Sanders Co., 1982, pp 142-148.

Light RW. Management of Spontaneous Pneumothorax. Am. Rev. Res. Dis. 1993; 148, 1: 245-248.

Light RW. Pneumothorax. In: Light RW, ed. Pleural Diseases. Philadelphia; Lea & Farbiger, 1990; 237-62.

Hematologic Disorders

Thomas Vovan, MD

Transfusion Reactions

I. **Acute hemolytic transfusion reaction**

    A. Transfusion reactions are rare and most commonly associated with ABO incompatibility, usually related to a clerical error. Early symptoms include sudden onset of anxiety, flushing, tachycardia, and hypotension. Chest and back pain, fever, and dyspnea are common.

    B. Life-threatening manifestations include vascular collapse (shock), renal failure, bronchospasm, and disseminated intravascular coagulation.

    C. Hemoglobinuria, and hemoglobinemia occurs because of intravascular red cell lysis.

    D. The direct antiglobulin test (direct Coombs test) is positive. The severity of reaction is usually related to the volume of RBCs infused.

    E. **Management**

        1. The transfusion should be discontinued immediately, and the unused donor blood and a sample of recipient's venous blood should be sent for retyping and repeat cross match, including a direct and indirect Coombs test.

        2. Urine analysis should be checked for free hemoglobin and centrifuged plasma for pink coloration (indicating free hemoglobin).

        3. Hypotension should be treated with normal saline. Vasopressors may be used if volume replacement alone is inadequate to maintain blood pressure.

        4. Maintain adequate renal perfusion with volume replacement. Furosemide may be used to maintain urine output after adequate volume replacement has been achieved.

        5. Monitor INR/PTT, platelets, fibrinogen, and fibrin degradation products for evidence of disseminated intravascular coagulation. Replace required clotting factors with fresh frozen plasma, platelets, and/or cryoprecipitate.

II. **Febrile transfusion reaction (nonhemolytic)**

    A. Febrile transfusion reactions occur in 0.5-3% of transfusions. It is most commonly seen in patients receiving multiple transfusions. Chills develop, followed by fever, usually during or within a few hours of transfusion. This reaction may be severe but is usually mild and self limited.

    B. **Management**

        1. Symptomatic and supportive care should be provided with acetaminophen and diphenhydramine. Meperidine 50 mg IV is useful in treating chills. A WBC filter should be used for the any subsequent transfusions.

        2. More serious transfusion reactions must be excluded (eg, acute hemolytic reaction or bacterial contamination of donor blood).

III. Transfusion-related noncardiogenic pulmonary edema

A. This reaction is characterized by sudden development of severe respiratory distress, associated with fever, chills, chest pain, and hypotension.

B. Chest radiograph demonstrates diffuse pulmonary edema. This reaction may be severe and life threatening but generally resolves within 48 hours.

C. **Management**

1. Treatment of pulmonary edema and hypoxemia may include mechanical ventilatory support and hemodynamic monitoring.

2. Diuretics are useful only if fluid overload is present. Use a WBC filter should be used for any subsequent transfusions.

Disseminated Intravascular Coagulation

I. Clinical manifestations

A. Disseminated intravascular coagulation (DIC) is manifest by generalized ecchymosis and petechiae, bleeding from peripheral IV sites, central catheters, surgical wounds, and oozing from gums.

B. Gastrointestinal and urinary tract bleeding are frequently encountered. Grayish discoloration or cyanosis of the distal fingers, toes, or ears may occur because of intravascular thrombosis. Large, sharply demarcated, ecchymotic areas may be seen as a result of thrombosis.

II. Diagnosis

A. Fibrin degradation products are the most sensitive screening test for DIC; however, no single laboratory parameter is diagnostic of DIC.

B. **Peripheral smear:** Evidence of microangiopathic hemolysis, with schistocytes and thrombocytopenia, is often present. A persistently normal platelet count nearly excludes the diagnosis of acute DIC.

C. **Coagulation studies:** INR, PTT, and thrombin time are generally prolonged. Fibrinogen levels are usually depleted (<150 mg/dL). Fibrin degradation products (>10 mg/dL) and D-dimer is elevated (>0.5 mg/dL).

III. Management of disseminated intravascular coagulation

A. The primary underlying precipitating condition (eg, sepsis) should be treated. Severe DIC with hypocoagulability may be treated with replacement of clotting factors. Hypercoagulability is managed with heparin.

B. Severe hemorrhage and shock is managed with fluids and red blood cell transfusions.

C. **If the patient is at high risk of bleeding or actively bleeding with DIC:** Replace fibrinogen with 10 units of cryoprecipitate. Replace clotting factors with 2-4 units of fresh frozen plasma. Replace platelets with platelet pheresis.

D. **If factor replacement therapy is transfused,** fibrinogen and platelet levels should be obtained 30-60 minutes post-transfusion and every 4-6 hours thereafter to determine the efficacy of therapy. Each unit of platelets should increase the platelet count by 5000-10,000/mcL. Each unit of cryoprecipitate should increase the fibrinogen level by 5-10 mg/dL.

E. **Heparin**

1. Indications for heparin include evidence of fibrin deposition (ie, dermal necrosis, acral ischemia, venous thromboembolism). Heparin is used when the coagulopathy is believed to be secondary to a retained, dead

fetus, amniotic fluid embolus, giant hemangioma, aortic aneurysm, solid tumors, or promyelocytic leukemia. Heparin is also used when clotting factors cannot be corrected with replacement therapy alone.

2. Heparin therapy is initiated at a relatively low dose (5-10 U/kg/hr) by continuous IV infusion without a bolus. Coagulation parameters must then be followed to guide therapy. The heparin dose may be increased by 2.5 U/kg/hr until the desired effect is achieved.

Thrombolytic-associated Bleeding

I. **Clinical presentation**: Post-fibrinolysis hemorrhage may present as a sudden neurologic deficit (intracranial bleeding), massive GI bleeding, progressive back pain accompanied by hypotension (retroperitoneal bleeding), or a gradual decline in hemoglobin without overt evidence of bleeding.

II. **Laboratory evaluation**
   A. Low fibrinogen (<100 mg/dL) and elevated fibrin degradation products confirm the presence of a lytic state. Elevated thrombin time and PTT may suggest a persistent lytic state; however, both are prolonged in the presence of heparin. Prolonged reptilase time identifies the persistent lytic state in the presence of heparin.
   B. Depleted fibrinogen in the fibrinolytic state will be reflected by an elevated PTT, thrombin time, or reptilase time. The post-transfusion fibrinogen level is a useful indicator of response to replacement therapy.
   C. The bleeding time may be a helpful guide to platelet replacement therapy if the patient has persistent bleeding despite factor replacement with cryoprecipitate and fresh frozen plasma.

III. **Management**
   A. Discontinue thrombolytics, aspirin, and heparin immediately, and consider protamine reversal of heparin and cryoprecipitate to replenish fibrinogen.
   B. Place two large-bore IV catheters for volume replacement. If possible, apply local pressure to bleeding sites. Blood specimens should be sent for INR/PTT, fibrinogen, and thrombin time. Reptilase time should be checked if the patient is also receiving heparin. Patient's blood should be typed and crossed because urgent transfusion may be needed.
   C. **Transfusion**
      1. Cryoprecipitate (10 units over 10 minutes) should be transfused to correct the lytic state. Transfusions may be repeated until the fibrinogen level is above 100 mg/dL or hemostasis is achieved. Cryoprecipitate is rich in fibrinogen and factor VIII.
      2. Fresh frozen plasma transfusion is also important for replacement of factor VIII and V. If bleeding persists after cryoprecipitate and FFP replacement, check a bleeding time and consider platelet transfusion if bleeding time is greater than 9 minutes. If bleeding time is less than 9 minutes, then antifibrinolytic drugs may be warranted.

D. Antifibrinolytic agents

1. Aminocaproic acid (EACA) inhibits the conversion of plasminogen to plasmin. It is used when replacement of blood products are not sufficient to attain hemostasis.
2. Loading dose: 5 g or 0.1 g/kg IV infused in 250 cc NS over 30-60 min, followed by continuous infusion at 0.5-2.0 g/h until bleeding is controlled. Use with caution in upper urinary tract bleeding because of the potential for obstruction.

References

Carr JM, McKinney M, McDonagh J: Diagnosis of Disseminated Intravascular Coagulation, Role of D-Dimer. Am J Clin Pathol 1989;91:280-287.

Feinstein DI: Treatment of Disseminated Intravascular Coagulation. Seminars in Thrombosis and Hemostasis. 1988;14:351-362.

Sane DC, Califf RM, Topol EJ, Stump DC, Mark DB, Greenberg CS: Bleeding during Thrombolytic Therapy for Acute Myocardial Infarction: Mechanisms and Management. Ann of Int Med. 1989;111:1010-1022.

Infectious Diseases

Guy Foster, MD
Farhad Mazdisnian, MD
Michael Krutzik, MD
Georgina Heal, MD

Bacterial Meningitis

The age group at greatest risk for acute bacterial meningitis (ABM) includes children between 1 and 24 months of age. Adults older than 60 years old account for 50% of all deaths related to meningitis.

I. **Clinical presentation**
   A. Eighty-five percent of patients with bacterial meningitis present with fever, headache, meningismus or nuchal rigidity, and altered mental status. Other common signs and symptoms include photophobia, vomiting, back pain, myalgias, diaphoresis, and malaise. Generalized seizures can occur in up to 40% of patients with ABM.
   B. Kernig's sign (resistance to extension of the leg while the hip is flexed) and Brudzinski's sign (involuntary flexion of the hip and knee when the patient's neck is abruptly flexed while laying supine) are observed in up to 50% of patients.
   C. About 50% of patients with N. meningitidis may present with an erythematous macular rash, which progresses to petechiae and purpura.

II. **Patient evaluation**
   A. **Computerized tomography (CT).** Patients who require CT prior to LP include those with focal neurologic findings, papilledema, focal seizures, or abnormalities on exam that suggest increased intracranial pressure. If bacterial meningitis is a strong consideration, and the decision is made to perform a CT prior to LP, two sets of blood cultures should be obtained and antibiotics should be administered before sending the patient for neuroimaging. Urine cultures may be helpful in the very young and very old.
   B. Blood cultures followed by antibiotic administration within 30 minutes of presentation is mandatory in all patients suspected of having bacterial meningitis.
   C. **Interpretation of lumbar puncture.** Examination of the CSF is mandatory for evaluation of meningitis.
   D. CSF, Gram's stain, and culture are positive in 70-85% of patients with ABM.

Cerebrospinal Fluid Parameters in Meningitis

	Normal	Bacterial	Viral	Fungal	TB	Para-menin-geal Focus or Abscess
WBC count (WBC/µL)	0-5	>1000	100-1000	100-500	100-500	10-1000
% PMN	0-15	90	<50	<50	<50	<50
% lymph		>50	>50	>80		
Glucose (mg/dL)	45-65	<40	45-65	30-45	30-45	45-65
CSF: blood glucose ratio	0.6	<0.4	0.6	<0.4	<0.4	0.6
Protein (mg/dL)	20-45	>150	50-100	100-500	100-500	>50
Opening pressure (cm H_2O)	6-20	>180 mm H_2O	NL or +	>180 mm H_2O	>180 mm H_2O	N/A

E. If the CSF parameters are nondiagnostic, or the patient has been treated with prior oral antibiotics, and, therefore, the Gram's stain and/or culture are likely to be negative, then latex agglutination (LA) may be helpful. The test has a variable sensitivity rate, ranging between 50-100%, and high specificity. Latex agglutination tests are available for H. influenza, Streptococcus pneumoniae, N. meningitidis, Escherichia coli K1, and S. agalactiae (Group B strep). CSF Cryptococcal antigen and India ink stain should be considered in patients who have HIV disease or HIV risk factors.

III. Treatment of acute bacterial meningitis

Antibiotic Choice Based on Age and Comorbid Medical Illness		
Age	**Organism**	**Antibiotic**
Neonate	E. coli, Group B strep, Listeria monocytogenes	Ampicillin and ceftriaxone or cefotaxime
1-3 months	S. pneumoniae, N. meningitidis, H. influenzae, S. agalactiae, Listeria, E. coli	Ceftriaxone or cefotaxime and vancomycin
3 months to 18 years	N. meningitidis, S. pneumoniae, H. influenzae	Ceftriaxone or cefotaxime and vancomycin
18-50 years	S. pneumoniae, N. meningitidis	Ceftriaxone or cefotaxime and vancomycin
Older than 50 years	N. meningitidis, S. pneumoniae Gram-negative bacilli, Listeria, Group B strep	Ampicillin and ceftriaxone or cefotaxime and vancomycin
Neurosurgery/head injury	S. aureus, S. epidermidis Diphtheroids, Gram-negative bacilli	Vancomycin and Ceftazidime
Immunosuppression	Listeria, Gram-negative bacilli, S. pneumoniae, N. meningitidis	Ampicillin and Ceftazidime (consider adding Vancomycin)
CSF shunt	S. aureus, Gram-negative bacilli	Vancomycin and Ceftazidime

Antibiotic Choice Based on Gram's Stain		
Stain Results	**Organism**	**Antibiotic**
Gram's (+) cocci	S. pneumoniae S. aureus, S. agalactiae (Group B)	Vancomycin and ceftriaxone or cefotaxime
Gram's (-) cocci	N. meningitidis	Penicillin G or chloramphenicol
Gram's (-) coccobacilli	H. influenzae	Third-generation cephalosporin

Stain Results	Organism	Antibiotic
Gram's (+) bacilli	Listeria monocytogenes	Ampicillin, Penicillin G + IV Gentamicin ± intrathecal gentamicin
Gram's (-) bacilli	E. coli, Klebsiella Serratia, Pseudomonas	Ceftazidime +/- aminoglycoside

Recommended Dosages of Antibiotics	
Antibiotic	**Dosage**
Ampicillin	2 g IV q4h
Cefotaxime	2 g IV q4-6h
Ceftazidime	2 g IV q8h
Ceftriaxone	2 g IV q12h
Chloramphenicol	0.5-1.0 gm IV q6h
Gentamicin	Load 2.0 mg/kg IV, then 1.5 mg/kg q8h
Nafcillin/Oxacillin	2 g IV q4h
Penicillin G	4 million units IV q4h
Rifampin	600 mg PO q24h
Trimethoprim-sulfamethoxazole	15 mg/kg IV q6h
Vancomycin	1.0-1.5 g IV q12h

A. In areas characterized by high resistance to penicillin, vancomycin plus a third-generation cephalosporin should be the first-line therapy. H. influenzae is usually adequately covered by a third-generation cephalosporin. The drug of choice for N. meningitidis is penicillin or ampicillin. Chloramphenicol should be used if the patient is allergic to penicillin. Aztreonam may be used for gram-negative bacilli, and trimethoprim-sulfamethoxazole may be used for Listeria.

B. In patients who are at risk for Listeria meningitis, ampicillin must be added to the regimen. S. agalactiae (Group B) is covered by ampicillin, and adding an aminoglycoside provides synergy. Pseudomonas and other Gram-negative bacilli should be treated with a broad spectrum third-generation cephalosporin (ceftazidime) plus an aminoglycoside. S. aureus may be covered by nafcillin or oxacillin. High-dose vancomycin (peak 35-40 mcg/mL) may be needed if the patient is at risk for methicillin-resistant S. aureus.

C. **Corticosteroids.** Audiologic and neurological sequelae in infants older than two months of age are markedly reduced by early administration of dexamethasone in patients with H. influenzae meningitis. Dexamethasone should be given at a dose of 0.15 mg/kg q6h IV for 2-4 days to children with suspected H. influenzae or pneumococcal meningitis. The dose should be given just prior to or with the initiation of antibiotics.

Pneumonia

Community-acquired pneumonia is the leading infectious cause of death and is the sixth-leading cause of death overall.

I. **Clinical diagnosis**
   A. **Symptoms** of pneumonia may include fever, chills, malaise and cough. Patients also may have pleurisy, dyspnea, or hemoptysis. Eighty percent of patients are febrile.
   B. **Physical exam findings** may include tachypnea, tachycardia, rales, rhonchi, bronchial breath sounds, and dullness to percussion over the involved area of lung.
   C. **Chest radiograph** usually shows infiltrates. The chest radiograph may reveal multilobar infiltrates, volume loss, or pleural effusion. The chest radiograph may be negative very early in the illness because of dehydration or severe neutropenia.
   D. **Additional testing** may include a complete blood count, pulse oximetry or arterial blood gas analysis.

II. **Laboratory evaluation**
   A. **Sputum for Gram stain and culture** should be obtained in hospitalized patients. In a patient who has had no prior antibiotic therapy, a high-quality specimen (>25 white blood cells and <5 epithelial cells/hpf) may help to direct initial therapy.
   B. **Blood cultures** are positive in 11% of cases, and cultures may identify a specific etiologic agent.
   C. **Serologic testing for HIV** is recommended in hospitalized patients between the ages of 15 and 54 years. **Urine antigen testing** for legionella is indicated in endemic areas for patients with serious pneumonia.

III. **Indications for hospitalization**
   A. Age >65years
   B. Unstable vital signs (heart rate >140 beats per minute, systolic blood pressure <90 mm Hg, respiratory rate >30 beats per minute)
   C. Altered mental status
   D. Hypoxemia (PO_2 <60 mm Hg)
   E. Severe underlying disease (lung disease, diabetes mellitus, liver disease, heart failure, renal failure)
   F. Immune compromise (HIV infection, cancer, corticosteroid use)
   G. Complicated pneumonia (extrapulmonary infection, meningitis, cavitation, multilobar involvement, sepsis, abscess, empyema, pleural effusion)
   H. Severe electrolyte, hematologic or metabolic abnormality (ie, sodium <130 mEq/L, hematocrit <30%, absolute neutrophil count <1,000/mm³, serum creatinine > 2.5 mg/dL)
   I. Failure to respond to outpatient treatment within 48 to 72 hours.

Pathogens Causing Community-Acquired Pneumonia	
More Common	**Less Common**
Streptococcus pneumoniae Haemophilus influenzae Moraxella catarrhalis Mycoplasma pneumoniae Chlamydia pneumoniae Legionella species Viruses Anaerobes (especially with aspiration)	Staphylococcus aureus Gram-negative bacilli Pneumocystis carinii Mycobacterium tuberculosis

IV. Treatment of community-acquired pneumonia

Recommended Empiric Drug Therapy for Patients with Community-Acquired Pneumonia		
Clinical Situation	**Primary Treatment**	**Alternative(s)**
Younger (<60 yr) outpatients without underlying disease	Macrolide antibiotics (azithromycin, clarithromycin, dirithromycin, or erythromycin)	Levofloxacin or doxycycline
Older (>60 yr) outpatients with underlying disease	Levofloxacin or cefuroxime or Trimethoprim-sulfamethoxazole Add vancomycin in severe, life-threatening pneumonias	Beta-lactamase inhibitor (with macrolide if legionella infection suspected)
Gross aspiration suspected	Clindamycin IV	Cefotetan, ampicillin/sulbactam

A. **Younger, otherwise healthy outpatients**
1. The most commonly identified organisms in this group are S pneumoniae, M pneumoniae, C pneumoniae, and respiratory viruses.
2. Erythromycin has excellent activity against most of the causal organisms in this group except H influenzae.
3. The newer macrolides, active against H influenzae (azithromycin [Zithromax] and clarithromycin [Biaxin]), are effective as empirical monotherapy for younger adults without underlying disease.

B. **Older outpatients with underlying disease**
1. The most common pathogens in this group are S pneumoniae, H influenzae, respiratory viruses, aerobic gram-negative bacilli, and S aureus. Agents such as M pneumoniae and C pneumoniae are not usually found in this group. Pseudomonas aeruginosa is rarely identified.

2. A second-generation cephalosporin (eg, cefuroxime [Ceftin]) is recommended for initial empirical treatment. Trimethoprim-sulfamethoxazole is an inexpensive alternative where pneumococcal resistance to not prevalent.

3. When legionella infection is suspected, initial therapy should include treatment with a macrolide antibiotic in addition to a beta-lactam/beta-lactamase inhibitor (amoxicillin clavulanate).

C. **Moderately ill, hospitalized patients**
   1. In addition to S pneumoniae and H influenzae, more virulent pathogens, such as S aureus, Legionella species, aerobic gram-negative bacilli (including P aeruginosa, and anaerobes), should be considered in patients requiring hospitalization.
   2. Hospitalized patients should receive an intravenous cephalosporin active against S pneumoniae and anaerobes (eg, cefuroxime, ceftriaxone [Rocephin], cefotaxime [Claforan]), or a beta-lactam/beta-lactamase inhibitor.
   3. **Nosocomial pneumonia** should be suspected in patients with recent hospitalization or nursing home status. Nosocomial pneumonia is most commonly caused by Pseudomonas or Staph aureus. Empiric therapy should consist of vancomycin and double pseudomonal coverage with a beta-lactam (cefepime, Zosyn, imipenem, ticarcillin, ceftazidime, cefoperazone) and an aminoglycoside (amikacin, gentamicin, tobramycin) or a quinolone (ciprofloxacin).
   4. When legionella is suspected (in endemic areas, cardiopulmonary disease, immune compromise), a macrolide should be added to the regimen. If legionella pneumonia is confirmed, rifampin (Rifadin) should be added to the macrolide.

Common Antimicrobial Agents for Community-Acquired Pneumonia in Adults		
Type	**Agent**	**Dosage**
Oral therapy		
Macrolides	Erythromycin Clarithromycin (Biaxin) Azithromycin (Zithromax)	500 mg PO qid 500 mg PO bid 500 mg PO on day 1, then 250 mg qd x 4 days
Beta-lactam/beta-lactamase inhibitor	Amoxicillin-clavulanate (Augmentin)	500 mg tid or 875 mg PO bid
Quinolones	Ciprofloxacin (Cipro) Levofloxacin (Levaquin) Ofloxacin (Floxin)	500 mg PO bid 500 mg PO qd 400 mg PO bid
Tetracycline	Doxycycline	100 m g PO bid
Sulfonamide	Trimethoprim-sulfamethoxazole	160 mg/800 mg (DS) PO bid

Type	Agent	Dosage
Intravenous Therapy		
Cephalosporins Second-generation	Cefuroxime (Kefurox, Zinacef)	0.75-1.5 g IV q8h
Third-generation (anti-Pseudomonas aeruginosa)	Ceftizoxime (Cefizox) Ceftazidime (Fortaz) Cefoperazone (Cefobid)	1-2 g IV q8h 1-2 g IV q8h 1-2 g IV q8h
Beta-lactam/beta- lactamase inhibitors	Ampicillin-sulbactam (Unasyn) Piperacillin/tazobactam (Zosyn) Ticarcillin-clavulanate (Timentin)	1.5 g IV q6h 3.375 g IV q6h 3.1 g IV q6h
Quinolones	Ciprofloxacin (Cipro) Levofloxacin (Levaquin) Ofloxacin (Floxin)	400 mg IV q12h 500 mg IV q24h 400 mg IV q12h
Aminoglycosides	Gentamicin Amikacin	Load 2.0 mg/kg IV, then 1.5 mg/kg q8h
Vancomycin	Vancomycin	1 gm IV q12h

D. Critically ill patients

1. S pneumoniae and Legionella species are the most commonly isolated pathogens, and aerobic gram-negative bacilli are identified with increasing frequency. M pneumoniae, respiratory viruses, and H influenzae are less commonly identified.

2. Erythromycin should be used along with an antipseudomonal agent (ceftazidime, imipenem-cilastatin [Primaxin], or ciprofloxacin [Cipro]). An aminoglycoside should be added for additional antipseudomonal activity until culture results are known.

3. Severe life-threatening community-acquired pneumonias should be treated with vancomycin empirically until culture results are known. Twenty-five percent of S. pneumoniae isolates are no longer susceptible to penicillin, and 9% are no longer susceptible to extended-spectrum cephalosporins.

4. Pneumonia caused by penicillin-resistant strains of S. pneumoniae should be treated with high-dose penicillin G (2-3 MU IV q4h), or cefotaxime (2 gm IV q8h), or ceftriaxone (2 gm IV q12h), or meropenem (Merrem) (500-1000 mg IV q8h), or vancomycin (Vancocin) (1 gm IV q12h).

5. H. influenzae and Moraxella catarrhalis often produce beta-lactamase enzymes, making these organisms resistant to penicillin and ampicillin. Infection with these pathogens is treated with a second-generation cephalosporin, beta-lactam/beta-lactamase inhibitor combination such as amoxicillin-clavulanate, azithromycin, or trimethoprim-sulfamethoxazole.

6. Most bacterial infections can be adequately treated with 10-14 days of antibiotic therapy. M pneumoniae and C pneumoniae infections require

treatment for up to 14 days. Legionella infections should be treated for a minimum of 14 days; immunocompromised patients require 21 days of therapy.

Pneumocystis Carinii Pneumonia

PCP is the most common life-threatening opportunistic infection occurring in patients with HIV disease. In the era of PCP prophylaxis and highly active antiretroviral therapy, the incidence of PCP is decreasing. The incidence of PCP has declined steadily from 50% in 1987 to 25% currently.

I. **Risk factors for Pneumocystis carinii pneumonia**
   A. Patients with CD4 counts of 200 cells/μL or less are 4.9 times more likely to develop PCP.
   B. Candidates for PCP prophylaxis include: patients with a prior history of PCP, patients with a CD4 cell count of less than 200 cells/μL, and HIV-infected patients with thrush or persistent fever.

II. **Clinical presentation**
   A. PCP usually presents with fever, dry cough, and shortness of breath or dyspnea on exertion with a gradual onset over several weeks. Tachypnea may be pronounced. Circumoral, acral, and mucous membrane cyanosis may be evident.
   B. **Laboratory findings**
      1. **Complete blood count and sedimentation rate** shows no characteristic pattern in patients with PCP. The serum LDH concentration is frequently increased.
      2. **Arterial blood gas** measurements generally show increases in $P(A-a)O_2$, although PaO_2 values vary widely depending on disease severity. Up to 25% of patients may have a PaO_2 of 80 mm Hg or above while breathing room air.
      3. **Pulmonary function tests.** Patients with PCP usually have a decreased diffusing capacity for carbon monoxide (DLCO).
   C. **Radiographic presentation**
      1. PCP in AIDS patients usually causes a diffuse interstitial infiltrate. High resolution computerized tomography (HRCT) may be helpful for those patients who have normal chest radiographic findings.
      2. Pneumatoceles (cavities, cysts, blebs, or bullae) and spontaneous pneumothoraces are common in patients with PCP.

III. **Laboratory diagnosis**
   A. **Sputum induction.** The least invasive means of establishing a specific diagnosis is the examination of sputum induced by inhalation of a 3-5% saline mist. The sensitivity of induced sputum examination for PCP is 74-77% and the negative predictive value is 58-64%. If the sputum tests negative, an invasive diagnostic procedure is required to confirm the diagnosis of PCP.
   B. **Transbronchial biopsy and bronchoalveolar lavage**. The sensitivity of transbronchial biopsy for PCP is 98%. The sensitivity of bronchoalveolar is 90%.
   C. **Open-lung biopsy** should be reserved for patients with progressive pulmonary disease in whom the less invasive procedures are nondiagnostic.

IV. Diagnostic algorithm

A. If the chest radiograph of a symptomatic patient appears normal, a DLCO should be performed. Patients with significant symptoms, a normal-appearing chest radiograph, and a normal DLCO should undergo high-resolution CT. Patients with abnormal findings at any of these steps should proceed to sputum induction or bronchoscopy. Sputum specimens collected by induction that reveal P. carinii should also be stained for acid-fast organisms and fungi, and the specimen should be cultured for mycobacteria and fungi.

B. Patients whose sputum examinations do not show P. carinii or another pathogen should undergo bronchoscopy.

C. Lavage fluid is stained for P. carinii, acid-fast organisms, and fungi. Also, lavage fluid is cultured for mycobacteria and fungi and inoculated onto cell culture for viral isolation. Touch imprints are made from tissue specimens and stained for P. carinii. Fluid is cultured for mycobacteria and fungi, and stained for P. carinii, acid-fast organisms, and fungi. If all procedures are nondiagnostic and the lung disease is progressive, open-lung biopsy may be considered.

V. Therapy and prophylaxis

A. **Trimethoprim-sulfamethoxazole DS (Bactrim DS, Septra DS)** is the recommended initial therapy for PCP. Dosage is 15-20 mg/kg/day of TMP IV divided q6h for 14-21 days. Adverse effects include rash (33%), elevation of liver enzymes (44%), nausea and vomiting (50%), anemia (40%), creatinine elevation (33%), and hyponatremia (94%).

B. **Pentamidine** is an alternative in patients who have adverse reactions or fail to respond to TMP-SMX. The dosage is 4 mg/kg/day IV for 14-21 days. Adverse effects include anemia (33%), creatinine elevation (60%), LFT elevation (63%), and hyponatremia (56%). Pancreatitis, hypoglycemia, and hyperglycemia are common side effects.

C. **Corticosteroids.** Adjunctive corticosteroid treatment is beneficial with anti-PCP therapy in patients with a partial pressure of oxygen (PaO_2) less than 70 mm Hg, (A-a)DO_2 greater than 35 mm Hg, or oxygen saturation less than 90% on room air. Contraindications include suspected tuberculosis or disseminated fungal infection. Treatment with methylprednisolone (SoluMedrol) should begin at the same time as anti-PCP therapy. The dosage is 30 mg IV q12h x 5 days, then 30 mg IV qd x 5 days, then 15 mg qd x 11 days **OR** prednisone, 40 mg twice daily for 5 days, then 40 mg daily for 5 days, and then 20 mg daily until day 21 of therapy.

VI. Prophylaxis

A. HIV-infected patients who have CD4 counts less than 200 cells/mcL should receive prophylaxis against PCP. If CD4 count increases to greater than 200 cells/mcL after receiving antiretroviral therapy, PCP prophylaxis can be safely discontinued.

B. **Trimethoprim-sulfamethoxazole** (once daily to three times weekly) is the preferred regimen for PCP prophylaxis.

C. **Dapsone** (100 mg daily or twice weekly) is a prophylactic regimen for patients who can not tolerate TMP-SMX.

D. **Aerosolized pentamidine (NebuPent)** 300 mg in 6 mL water nebulized over 20 min q4 weeks is another alternative.

Antiretroviral Therapy and Opportunistic Infections in AIDS

I. **Antiretroviral therapy**
   A. A combination of three agents is recommended as initial therapy. The preferred options are 2 nucleosides plus 1 protease inhibitor or 1 non-nucleoside. Alternative options are 2 protease inhibitors plus 1 nucleoside or 1 non-nucleoside. Combinations of 1 nucleoside, 1 non-nucleoside, and 1 protease inhibitor are also effective.
   B. **Nucleoside analogs**
      1. Abacavir (Ziagen) 300 mg PO bid [300 mg].
      2. Didanosine (Videx) 200 mg PO bid [chewable tabs: 25, 50, 100, 150 mg]; oral ulcers discourage common usage.
      3. Lamivudine (Epivir) 150 mg PO bid [tab: 150 mg].
      4. Stavudine (Zerit) 40 mg PO bid [cap: 15, 20, 30, 40 mg].
      5. Zalcitabine (Hivid) 0.75 mg PO tid [tab: 0.375, 0.75 mg].
      6. Zidovudine (Retrovir, AZT) 200 mg PO tid or 300 mg PO bid [cap: 100, 300 mg].
      7. Zidovudine 300 mg/lamivudine 150 mg (Combivir) 1 tab PO bid.
   C. **Protease inhibitors**
      1. Amprenavir (Agenerase) 1200 mg PO bid [50, 150 mg]
      2. Indinavir (Crixivan) 800 mg PO tid [cap: 200, 400 mg].
      3. Nelfinavir (Viracept) 750 mg PO tid [tab: 250 mg]
      4. Ritonavir (Norvir) 600 mg PO bid [cap: 100 mg].
      5. Saquinavir (Invirase) 600 mg PO tid [cap: 200 mg].
   D. **Non-nucleoside analogs**
      1. Delavirdine (Rescriptor) 400 mg PO tid [tab: 100 mg]
      2. Efavirenz (Sustiva) 600 mg qhs [50, 100, 200 mg]
      3. Nevirapine (Viramune) 200 mg PO bid [tab: 200 mg]
II. **Oral candidiasis**
   A. Fluconazole (Diflucan), acute: 200 mg PO x 1, then 100 mg qd x 5 days
   OR
   B. Ketoconazole (Nizoral), acute: 400 mg po qd 1-2 weeks or until resolved
   OR
   C. Clotrimazole (Mycelex) troches 10 mg dissolved slowly in mouth 5 times/d.
III. **Candida esophagitis**
   A. Fluconazole (Diflucan) 200 mg PO x 1, then 100 mg PO qd until improved.
   B. Ketoconazole (Nizoral) 200 mg po bid.
IV. **Primary or recurrent mucocutaneous HSV**. Acyclovir (Zovirax), 200-400 mg PO 5 times a day for 10 days, or 5 mg/kg IV q8h; or in cases of acyclovir resistance, foscarnet 40 mg/kg IV q8h for 21 days.
V. **Herpes simplex encephalitis**. Acyclovir 10 mg/kg IV q8h x 10-21 days.
VI. **Herpes varicella zoster**
   A. Acyclovir (Zovirax) 10 mg/kg IV over 60 min q8h **OR**
   B. Valacyclovir (Valtrex) 1000 mg PO tid x 7 days [caplet: 500 mg].
VII. **Cytomegalovirus infections**
   A. Ganciclovir (Cytovene) 5 mg/kg IV (dilute in 100 mL D5W over 60 min) q12h x 14-21 days (concurrent use with zidovudine increases hematological toxicity).

    B. Suppressive treatment for CMV: Ganciclovir (Cytovene) 5 mg/kg IV qd, or 6 mg/kg IV 5 times/wk, or 1000 mg orally tid with food.

VIII. Toxoplasmosis

    A. Pyrimethamine 200 mg PO loading dose, then 50-75 mg qd plus leucovorin calcium (folinic acid) 10-20 mg PO qd for 6-8 weeks for acute therapy **AND**

    B. Sulfadiazine (1.0-1.5 gm PO q6h) or clindamycin 450 mg PO qid/600-900 mg IV q6h.

    C. Suppressive treatment for toxoplasmosis

        1. Pyrimethamine 25-50 mg PO qd with or without sulfadiazine 0.5-1.0 gm PO q6h; and folinic acid 5-10 mg PO qd **OR**

        2. Pyrimethamine 50 mg PO qd; and clindamycin 300 mg PO q6h; and folinic acid 5-10 mg PO qd.

IX. Cryptococcus neoformans meningitis

    A. Amphotericin B at 0.7 mg/kg/d IV for 14 days or until clinically stable, followed by fluconazole (Diflucan) 400 mg qd to complete 10 weeks of therapy, followed by suppressive therapy with fluconazole (Diflucan) 200 mg PO qd indefinitely.

    B. Amphotericin B lipid complex (Abelcet) may be used in place of non-liposomal amphotericin B if the patient is intolerant to non-liposomal amphotericin B. The dosage is 5 mg/kg IV q24h.

X. Active tuberculosis

    A. Isoniazid (INH) 300 mg PO qd; and rifabutin 300 mg PO qd; and pyrazinamide 15-25 mg/kg PO qd (500 mg PO bid-tid); and ethambutol 15-25 mg/kg PO qd (400 mg PO bid-tid).

    B. All four drugs are continued for 2 months; isoniazid and rifabutin (depending on susceptibility testing) are continued for a period of at least 9 months and at least 6 months after the last negative cultures.

    C. Pyridoxine (vitamin B6) 50 mg PO qd, concurrent with INH.

XI. Disseminated mycobacterium avium complex (MAC)

    A. Azithromycin (Zithromax) 500-1000 mg PO qd or clarithromycin (Biaxin) 500 mg PO bid; **AND**

    B. Ethambutol 15-25 mg/kg PO qd (400 mg bid-tid) **AND**

    C. Rifabutin 300 mg/d (two 150 mg tablets qd).

    D. Prophylaxis for MAC

        1. Clarithromycin (Biaxin) 500 mg PO bid **OR**

        2. Rifabutin (Mycobutin) 300 mg PO qd or 150 mg PO bid.

XII. Disseminated coccidioidomycosis

    A. Amphotericin B (Fungizone) 0.8 mg/kg IV qd **OR**

    B. Amphotericin B lipid complex (Abelcet) 5 mg/kg IV q24h **OR**

    C. Fluconazole (Diflucan) 400-800 mg PO or IV qd.

XIII. Disseminated histoplasmosis

    A. Amphotericin B (Fungizone) 0.5-0.8 mg/kg IV qd, until total dose 15 mg/kg **OR**

    B. Amphotericin B lipid complex (Abelcet) 5 mg/kg IV q24h **OR**

    C. Itraconazole (Sporanox) 200 mg PO bid.

    D. Suppressive treatment for histoplasmosis: Itraconazole (Sporanox) 200 mg PO bid.

Sepsis

Sepsis is the most common cause of death in medical and surgical ICUs. Mortality ranges from 20-60%. The systemic inflammatory response syndrome (SIRS) is an inflammatory response that is a manifestation of both sepsis and the inflammatory response that results from trauma or burns. The term "sepsis" is reserved for patients who have SIRS attributable to infection.

I. **Pathophysiology**
A. Although gram-negative bacteremia is commonly found in patients with sepsis, gram-positive infection may affect 30-40% of patients. Fungal, viral and parasitic infections are usually encountered in immunocompromised patients.

Defining sepsis and related disorders	
Term	**Definition**
Systemic inflammatory response syndrome (SIRS)	The systemic inflammatory response to a severe clinical insult manifested by ≥2 of the following conditions: Temperature >38°C or <36°C, heart rate >90 beats/min, respiratory rate >20 breaths/min or $PaCO_2$ <32 mm Hg, white blood cell count >12,000 cells/mm^3, <4000 cells/mm^3, or >10% band cells
Sepsis	The presence of SIRS caused by an infectious process; sepsis is considered severe if hypotension or systemic manifestations of hypoperfusion (lactic acidosis, oliguria, change in mental status) is present.
Septic shock	Sepsis-induced hypotension despite adequate fluid resuscitation, along with the presence of perfusion abnormalities that may induce lactic acidosis, oliguria, or an alteration in mental status.
Multiple organ dysfunction syndrome (MODS)	The presence of altered organ function in an acutely ill patient such that homeostasis cannot be maintained without intervention

B. Sources of bacteremia leading to sepsis include the urinary, respiratory and GI tracts, and skin and soft tissues (including catheter sites). The source of bacteremia is unknown in 30% of patients.
C. Escherichia coli is the most frequently encountered gram-negative organism, followed by Klebsiella, Enterobacter, Serratia, Pseudomonas, Proteus, Providencia, and Bacteroides species. Up to 16% of sepsis cases are polymicrobic.
D. Gram-positive organisms, including Staphylococcus aureus and Staphylococcus epidermidis, are associated with catheter or line-related infections.

II. **Clinical evaluation**
A. Although fever is the most common sign of sepsis, normal body temperatures and hypothermia are common in the elderly. Tachypnea and/or hyperventilation with respiratory alkalosis may occur before the

onset of fever or leukocytosis. Other common clinical signs of systemic inflammation or impaired organ perfusion include altered mentation, oliguria, and tachycardia.

B. In the early stages of sepsis, tachycardia is associated with increased cardiac output; peripheral vasodilation; and a warm, well-perfused appearance. As shock progresses, vascular resistance continues to fall, hypotension ensues and myocardial depression results in decreased cardiac output. During the later stages of septic shock, vasoconstriction and cold extremities develop.

C. **Laboratory findings.** In the early stages of sepsis, arterial blood gas measurements usually reveal respiratory alkalosis. As shock ensues, metabolic acidosis becomes apparent. Hypoxemia is common.

Manifestations of Sepsis	
Clinical features	**Laboratory findings**
Temperature instability	Respiratory alkaloses
Tachypnea	Hypoxemia
Hyperventilation	Increased serum lactate levels
Altered mental status	Leukocytosis and increased neutrophil
Oliguria	concentration
Tachycardia	Eosinopenia
Peripheral vasodilation	Thrombocytopenia
	Anemia
	Proteinuria
	Mildly elevated serum bilirubin levels

D. **Hemodynamics**

1. The hallmark of early septic shock is a dramatic drop in systemic vascular resistance, resulting in a decrease in blood pressure.

2. Cardiac output rises in response to the fall in systemic blood pressure. This is referred to as the "hyperdynamic state" in sepsis. Shock results if the increase in cardiac output is insufficient to maintain blood pressure. Diminished cardiac output may occur as systemic blood pressure falls.

III. **Treatment of sepsis**

A. **Resuscitation.** During the initial resuscitation of a hypotensive patient with sepsis, large volumes of IV fluid should be given. Initial resuscitation may require 4-6 L of crystalloid. Fluid infusion volumes should be titrated to obtain a pulmonary capillary wedge pressure of 10-20 mm Hg. Other indices of organ perfusion include oxygen delivery, serum lactate levels, arterial blood pressure, and urinary output.

B. **Vasopressor and inotropic therapy** is necessary if hypotension persists despite aggressive fluid resuscitation.

1. **Dopamine** is a first-line agent for sepsis-associated hypotension. Begin with 5 μg/kg/min and titrate the dosage to the desired blood pressure response, usually a systolic blood pressure of greater than 90 mm Hg.

2. **Norepinephrine or phenylephrine infusions** may be used if hypotension persists despite high dosages of dopamine (20 μg/kg/min), or if dopamine causes excessive tachycardia. These agents have alpha-adrenergic effects, causing peripheral vasoconstriction and increased the mean arterial pressure.

3. **Dobutamine** can be added to increase cardiac output through its beta-adrenergic inotropic effects.
4. **Epinephrine** has both alpha- and beta-adrenergic properties. Epinephrine may be added if hypotension persists despite maximum doses of dopamine and norepinephrine.

C. **Activated protein C** is a vitamin K-dependent plasma protein which limits coagulation and augments fibrinolysis. In severe sepsis, activated protein C (24 mcg/kg/hr for 96 hours) has been shown to decrease mortality from 30.8 to 24.7%. It should not be used in patients with thrombocytopenia, coagulopathy, recent surgery or recent hemorrhage because it increases the risk of bleeding.

Vasoactive and Inotropic Drugs	
Agent	**Dosage**
Dopamine	**Inotropic Dose:** 5-10 mcg/kg/min **Vasoconstricting Dose:** 10-20 mcg/kg/min
Dobutamine	**Inotropic:** 5-10 mcg/kg/min **Vasodilator:** 15-20 mcg/kg/min
Norepinephrine	**Vasoconstricting dose:** 2-8 mcg/min
Phenylephrine	**Vasoconstricting dose:** 20-200 mcg/min
Epinephrine	**Vasoconstricting dose:** 1-8 mcg/min

A. **Diagnosis and management infection**
1. **Initial treatment of life-threatening sepsis** usually consists of a third-generation cephalosporin (ceftazidime, cefotaxime, ceftizoxime), piperacillin/tazobactam, or imipenem. An aminoglycoside (gentamicin, tobramycin, or amikacin) should also be included. Antipseudomonal coverage is important for hospital- or institutional-acquired infections. Appropriate choices include an antipseudomonal penicillin, cephalosporin, or an aminoglycoside.
2. **Methicillin-resistant staphylococci.** If line sepsis or an infected implanted device is a possibility, vancomycin should be added to the regimen to cover for methicillin-resistant Staph aureus and methicillin-resistant Staph epidermidis.
3. **Intra-abdominal or pelvic infections** are likely to involve anaerobes; therefore, treatment should include either piperacillin/tazobactam (Zosyn), imipenem (Primaxin), or meropenem (Merrem). Alternatively, metronidazole with an aminoglycoside and ampicillin may be initiated.
4. **Biliary tract infections.** When the source of bacteremia is the biliary tract, piperacillin/tazobactam (Zosyn) or cefoperazone (Cefobid) may be used. An aminoglycoside plus clindamycin is an alternative.

Dosages of antibiotics used in sepsis	
Agent	**Dosage**
Cefotaxime (Claforan)	2 gm q4-6h
Ceftizoxime (Cefizox)	2 gm IV q8h
Cefoxitin (Mefoxin)	2 gm q6h
Cefotetan (Cefotan)	2 gm IV q12h
Ceftazidime (Fortaz)	2 g IV q8h
Ticarcillin/clavulanate (Timentin)	3.1 gm IV q4-6h (200-300 mg/kg/d)
Ampicillin/sulbactam (Unasyn)	3.0 gm IV q6h
Piperacillin/tazobactam (Zosyn)	3.375-4.5 gm IV q6h
Piperacillin, ticarcillin, mezlocillin	3 gm IV q4-6h
Meropenem (Merrem)	1 gm IV q8h
Imipenem/cilastatin (Primaxin)	1.0 gm IV q6h
Gentamicin or tobramycin	2 mg/kg IV loading dose, then 1.7 mg/kg IV q8h
Amikacin (Amikin)	7.5 mg/kg IV loading dose, then 5 mg/kg IV q8h
Vancomycin	1 gm IV q12h
Metronidazole (Flagyl)	500 mg IV q6-8h
Linezolid (Zyvox)	600 mg IV/PO q12h
Quinupristin/dalfopristin (Synercid)	7.5 mg/kg IV q8h

5. **Vancomycin-resistant enterococcus (VRE):** An increasing number of enterococcal strains are resistant to ampicillin and gentamicin. The incidence of vancomycin-resistant enterococcus (VRE) is rapidly increasing.
   a. **Linezolid (Zyvox)** is an oral or parenteral agent active against vancomycin-resistant enterococci, including E. faecium and E. faecalis. Linezolid is also active against methicillin-resistant staphylococcus aureus.
   b. **Quinupristin/dalfopristin (Synercid)** is a parenteral agent active against strains of vancomycin-resistant enterococcus faecium, but not enterococcus faecalis. Most strains of VRE are enterococcus faecium.

Peritonitis

I. Acute Peritonitis

A. Acute peritonitis is inflammation of the peritoneum or peritoneal fluid from bacteria or intestinal contents in the peritoneal cavity. Secondary peritonitis results from perforation of a viscus caused by acute appendicitis or diverticulitis, perforation of an ulcer, or trauma. Primary peritonitis refers to peritonitis arising without a recognizable preceding cause. Tertiary peritonitis consists of persistent intra-abdominal sepsis without a discrete focus of infection, usually occurring after surgical treatment of peritonitis.

B. Clinical features

1. Acute peritonitis presents with abdominal pain, abdominal tenderness, and the absence of bowel sounds. Severe, sudden-onset abdominal pain suggests a ruptured viscus. Signs of peritoneal irritation include abdominal tenderness, rebound tenderness, and abdominal rigidity.

2. In severe cases, fever, hypotension, tachycardia, and acidosis may occur. Spontaneous bacterial peritonitis arising from ascites will often present with only subtle signs.

C. Diagnosis

1. **Plain abdominal radiographs and a chest x-ray** may detect free air in the abdominal cavity caused by a perforated viscus. CT and/or ultrasonography can identify the presence of free fluid or an abscess.

2. **Paracentesis**

   a. **Tube 1** - Cell count and differential (1-2 mL, EDTA purple top tube)

   b. **Tube 2** - Gram stain of sediment; C&S, AFB, fungal C&S (3-4 mL); inject 10-20 mL into anaerobic and aerobic culture bottle at the bedside.

   c. **Tube 3** - Glucose, protein, albumin, LDH, triglyceride, specific gravity, amylase, (2-3 mL, red top tube). Serum/fluid albumin gradient should be determined.

   d. **Syringe** - pH (3 mL).

D. Treatment of acute peritonitis

1. Resuscitation with intravenous fluids and correction of metabolic and electrolyte disturbances are the initial steps. Laparotomy is a cornerstone of therapy for secondary or tertiary acute peritonitis.

2. Broad-spectrum systemic antibiotics are critical to cover bowel flora, including anaerobic species.

3. **Mild to moderate infection (community-acquired)**

   a. Cefotetan (Cefotan) 1-2 gm IV q12h **OR**

   b. Ampicillin/sulbactam (Unasyn) 3.0 gm IV q6h

   c. Ticarcillin/clavulanate (Timentin) 3.1 gm IV q6h

4. **Severe infection (hospital-acquired)**

   a. Cefepime (Maxipime) 2 gm IV q12h and metronidazole (Flagyl) 500 mg IV q6h **OR**

   b. Piperacillin/tazobactam (Zosyn) 3.375 gm IV q6h **OR**

   c. Imipenem/cilastatin (Primaxin) 1 g IV q6h **OR**

   d. Ciprofloxacin (Cipro) 400 mg IV q12h and clindamycin 600 mg IV q8h **OR**

> e. Gentamicin or tobramycin 100-120 mg (1.5 mg/kg); then 80 mg IV q8h (3-5 mg/kg/d) and metronidazole (Flagyl) 500 mg IV q6h.

II. Spontaneous bacterial peritonitis

A. SBP, which has no obvious precipitating cause, occurs almost exclusively in cirrhotic patients

B. Diagnosis

1. Spontaneous bacterial peritonitis is diagnosed by paracentesis in which the ascitic fluid is found to have 250 or more polymorphonuclear (PMN) cells per cubic millimeter.

C. Therapy

1. Antibiotics are the cornerstone of managing SBP, and laparotomy has no place in therapy for SBP, unless perforation is present. Three to 5 days of intravenous treatment with broad-spectrum antibiotics is usually adequate, at which time efficacy can be determined by estimating the ascitic fluid PMN cell count.

2. **Option 1:**

   a. Cefotaxime (Claforan) 2 gm IV q4-6h

3. **Option 2:**

   a. Ticarcillin/clavulanate (Timentin) 3.1 gm IV q6h **OR**

   b. Piperacillin/tazobactam (Zosyn) 3.375 gm IV q6h or 4.5 gm IV q8h.

4. **Option 3 if extended-spectrum beta-lactamase (ESBL):**

   a. Imipenem/cilastatin (Primaxin) 1.0 gm IV q6h. **OR**

   b. Ciprofloxacin (Cipro) 400 mg IV q12h **OR**

   c. Levofloxacin (Levaquin) 500 mg IV q24h.

References

Drugs for HIV Infection. The Medical letter 2000; 42:1-6.

Preface to the 1997 USPHS/IDSA Guidelines for the Prevention of Opportunistic Infections in Persons Infected with HIV.

1997 Guidelines for the Use of Antimicrobial Agents in Neutropenic Patients with Unexplained Fever. Clinical Infectious Diseases 1997; 25:551-73

Hughes W.T. Opportunistic Infections in AIDS Patients. Opportunistic Infections 95:81-93, 1994

Lane HCLaughon B.E. Falloon J., et. al. Recent Advances in the Management of AIDS-related Opportunistic Infections. Ann. Intern. Med. 120:945-955, 1994.

Tunkel A.R, Wispelway B, Scheld W.N: Bacterial meningitis; Recent advances in pathophysiology and treatment. Ann Int Med 112:610,1990.

Pachon J, et al: Severe community acquired pneumonia. Am Rev Respir Dis 142:36973, 1990

Whittman, DH. Management of Secondary Peritonitis. Annals of Surgery. 1996; 224 (1): 10-18.

Bernard, GR, et al. Efficacy and Safety of Recombinant Human Activated Protein C for Severe Sepsis. NEJM. 2001; Vol 334, No 10: 699-709.

Gastroenterology

Michael Krutzik, MD
H.L. Daneschvar, MD
S.E. Wilson, MD
Roham T. Zamanian, MD

Upper Gastrointestinal Bleeding

I. **Clinical evaluation**
   A. Initial evaluation of upper GI bleeding should estimate the severity, duration, location, and cause of bleeding. A history of bleeding occurring after forceful vomiting suggests Mallory-Weiss Syndrome.
   B. Abdominal pain, melena, hematochezia (bright red blood per rectum), history of peptic ulcer, cirrhosis or prior bleeding episodes may be present.
   C. **Precipitating factors.** Use of aspirin, nonsteroidal anti-inflammatory drugs, alcohol, or anticoagulants should be sought.

II. **Physical examination**
   A. **General:** Pallor and shallow, rapid respirations may be present; tachycardia indicates a 10% blood volume loss. Postural hypotension (increase in pulse of 20 and a systolic blood pressure fall of 10-15 mmHg), indicates a 20-30% loss.
   B. **Skin:** Delayed capillary refill and stigmata of liver disease (jaundice, spider angiomas, parotid gland hypertrophy) should be sought.
   C. **Abdomen:** Scars, tenderness, masses, hepatomegaly, and dilated abdominal veins should be evaluated. Stool gross or occult blood should be checked.

III. **Laboratory evaluation:** CBC, SMA 12, liver function tests, amylase, INR/PTT, type and cross for pRBC, FFP, EKG.

IV. **Differential diagnosis of upper bleeding:** Peptic ulcer, gastritis, esophageal varices, Mallory-Weiss tear, esophagitis, swallowed blood from epistaxis, malignancy (esophageal, gastric), angiodysplasias, aorto-enteric fistula, hematobilia.

V. **Management of upper gastrointestinal bleeding**
   A. If the bleeding appears to have stopped or has significantly slowed, medical therapy with H2 blockers and saline lavage is usually all that is required.
   B. Two 14- to16-gauge IV lines should be placed. Normal saline solution should be infused until blood is ready, then transfuse 2-6 units of pRBCs as fast as possible. An estimate of blood transfusion requirement should be based on the blood loss rate and vital signs (typically 2-6 units are needed).
   C. A large bore nasogastric tube should be placed, followed by lavage with 2 L of room temperature tap water. The tube should then be connected to low intermittent suction, and the lavage should be repeated hourly. The NG tube may be removed when bleeding is no longer active.
   D. Oxygen is administered by nasal cannula, guided by pulse oximetry. Urine output should be monitored.
   E. Serial hematocrits should be checked and maintained greater than 30%.

    F. Coagulopathy should be assessed and corrected with fresh frozen plasma, vitamin K, cryoprecipitate, and platelets.

    G. Definitive diagnosis requires upper endoscopy, at which time electrocoagulation, banding, and/or local injection of vasoconstrictors at bleeding sites may be completed.

    H. Surgical consultation should be requested in unstable patients or patients who require more than 6 units of pRBCs.

VI. Mallory-Weiss syndrome

    A. This disorder is defined as a mucosal tear at the gastroesophageal junction following forceful retching and vomiting.

    B. Treatment is supportive, and the majority of patients stop bleeding spontaneously. Endoscopic coagulation or operative suturing may rarely be necessary.

VII. Acute medical treatment of peptic ulcer disease

    A. Ranitidine (Zantac) 50 mg IV bolus, then continuous infusion at 6.25-12.5 mg/h [150-300 mg in 250 mL D5W over 24h (11 cc/h)], or 50 mg IV q6-8h **OR**

    B. Cimetidine (Tagamet) 300 mg IV bolus, then continuous infusion at 37.5-50 mg/h (900 mg in 250 mL D5W over 24h), or 300 mg IV q6-8h **OR**

    C. Famotidine (Pepcid) 20 mg IV q12h.

Variceal Bleeding

Hemorrhage from esophageal and gastric varices usually occurs as a complication of chronic liver disease.

I. Clinical evaluation

    A. Variceal bleeding should be considered in any patient who presents with significant upper gastrointestinal bleeding. Signs of cirrhosis may include spider angiomas, palmar erythema, leukonychia, clubbing, parotid enlargement, and Dupuytren's contracture. Jaundice, lower extremity edema and ascites are indicative of decompensated liver disease.

    B. The severity of the bleeding episode can be assessed on the basis of orthostatic changes (eg, resting tachycardia, postural hypotension), which indicates one-third or more of blood volume loss.

    C. If the patient's sensorium is altered because of hepatic encephalopathy, the risk of aspiration mandates endotracheal intubation. Placement of a large-caliber nasogastric tube (22 F or 24 F) permits lavage for removal of blood and clots in preparation for endoscopy.

    D. Nasogastric lavage should be performed with tap water, because saline may contribute to retention of sodium and water.

II. Resuscitation

    A. Blood should be replaced as soon as possible. While blood for transfusion is being made available, intravascular volume should be replenished with normal saline solution.

    B. Once euvolemia is established, the intravenous infusion should be changed to solutions with a lower sodium content (5% dextrose with ½ or ¼ normal saline).

    C. Fresh frozen plasma is administered to patients who have been given massive transfusions. Each 3 units of PRBC should be accompanied by $CaCL_2$ 1 gm IV over 30 min.

D. Blood should be transfused to maintain a hematocrit of at least 30%. Serial hematocrit estimations should be obtained during continued bleeding.

III. Treatment of variceal hemorrhage

A. Pharmacologic agents

1. **Octreotide (Sandostatin)** 50 mcg IV over 5-10 min, followed by 50 mcg/h for 48 hours (1200 mcg in 250 mL D5W). Octreotide is a somatostatin analog, which is beneficial in controlling hemorrhage.

2. **Vasopressin (Pitressin)**, a posterior pituitary hormone, causes splanchnic arteriolar vasoconstriction and reduction in portal pressure.

    a. Dosage is 20 units IV over 20-30 min, then 0.2-0.4 units/minute (100 U in 250 mL D5W).

    b. Concomitant use of IV nitroglycerin paste (1 inch q6h) mitigates the vasoconstrictor effects of vasopressin on the myocardial and splanchnic circulations.

B. Tamponade devices

1. Bleeding from varices may temporarily be reduced with tamponade balloon tubes. However, the benefit is temporary, and prolonged tamponade causes severe esophageal ulceration and has a high rebleeding rate. The Linton-Nachlas tube has a gastric balloon and several ports in the esophageal component. The tube is kept in place for 6-12 hours while preparations for endoscopic or radiologic treatment are being made.

C. Endoscopic management of bleeding varices

1. **Endoscopic sclerotherapy** involves injection of a sclerosant into varices. The success of the treatment is enhanced by a second sclerotherapy treatment.

2. **Endoscopic variceal ligation** involves placement of tiny rubber bands on varices during endoscopy. Ligation is associated with fewer complications than sclerotherapy, but both have comparable efficacy.

D. Surgery

1. Portal-systemic shunt surgery is the most definitive therapy for bleeding varices. However, the procedures have a 30-40% rate of hepatic encephalopathy, and there is only a slight survival advantage over medical treatment.

2. Shunts that preserve portal blood flow are preferred, such as the distal splenorenal and the small-diameter portacaval H-graft shunts.

E. Transjugular intrahepatic portacaval shunt (TIPS)

1. Under fluoroscopy, a needle is advanced into the liver through the internal jugular and hepatic veins, and inserted into a large branch of the portal vein. A balloon is then used to enlarge the track to permit the placement of a stent.

2. Encephalopathy occurs in about 35% of patients, and there is a significant risk of shunt thrombosis or stenosis.

IV. Approach to treatment of variceal hemorrhage

A. Patients initially should be given octreotide (Sandostatin) or vasopressin infusion plus nitroglycerin while awaiting endoscopic treatment.

B. If varices are large, endoscopic ligation is preferred. If there is active bleeding from a spurting varix, sclerotherapy is best.

C. Failure of endoscopic therapy warrants the use of a portal-systemic shunt. Liver transplantation should be considered in poor-risk patients and when other therapies fail.

Lower Gastrointestinal Bleeding

H.L. Daneschvar, MD
S.E. Wilson, MD

The spontaneous remission rates for lower gastrointestinal bleeding is 80 percent. No source of bleeding can be identified in 12 percent of patients, and bleeding is recurrent in 25 percent. Bleeding has usually ceased by the time the patient presents to the emergency room.

I. **Clinical evaluation**
  A. The severity of blood loss and hemodynamic status should be assessed immediately. Initial management consists of resuscitation with crystalloid solutions (lactated Ringers solution) and blood products if necessary.
  B. The duration and quantity of bleeding should be assessed; however, the duration of bleeding is often underestimated.
  C. **Risk factors** that may have contributed to the bleeding include and nonsteroidal anti-inflammatory drugs, anticoagulants, colonic diverticulitis, renal failure, coagulopathy, colonic polyps, and hemorrhoids. Patients may have a prior history of hemorrhoids, diverticulosis, inflammatory bowel disease, peptic ulcer, gastritis, cirrhosis, or esophageal varices.
  D. **Hematochezia.** Bright red or maroon output per rectum suggests a lower GI source; however 12 to 20% of patients with an upper GI bleed may have hematochezia as a result of rapid blood loss.
  E. **Melena.** Sticky, black, foul-smelling stools suggest a source proximal to the ligament of Treitz, but Melena can also result from bleeding in the small intestine or proximal colon.
  F. **Change in stool caliber, anorexia, weight loss and malaise** are suggestive of malignancy.
  G. Clinical findings
    1. **Abdominal pain** may result from ischemic bowel, inflammatory bowel disease, or a ruptured aneurysm.
    2. **Painless massive bleeding** suggests vascular bleeding from diverticula, angiodysplasia, or hemorrhoids.
    3. **Bloody diarrhea** suggests inflammatory bowel disease or an infectious origin.
    4. **Bleeding with rectal pain** is seen with anal fissures, hemorrhoids, and rectal ulcers.
    5. **Chronic constipation** suggests hemorrhoidal bleeding. New onset of constipation or thin stools suggests a left sided colonic malignancy.
    6. **Blood on the toilet paper** or dripping into the toilet water suggests a perianal source of bleeding, such as hemorrhoids or an anal fissure.
    7. **Blood coating** the outside of stools suggests a lesion in the anal canal.
    8. **Blood streaking** or mixed in with the stool may results from polyps or a malignancy in the descending colon.
    9. **Maroon colored stools** often indicate small bowel and proximal colon bleeding.
II. **Physical examination**
  A. **Postural hypotension** indicates a 20% blood volume loss, whereas, overt signs of shock (pallor, hypotension, tachycardia) indicates a 30 to 40 percent blood loss.

   B. **The skin** may be cool and pale with delayed refill if bleeding has been significant.

   C. **Stigmata of liver disease**, including jaundice, caput medusae, gynecomastia and palmar erythema, should be sought because patients with these findings frequently have GI bleeding.

III. **Differential diagnosis of lower GI bleeding**

   A. **Angiodysplasia** and diverticular disease of the right colon accounts for the vast majority of episodes of acute lower GI bleeding. Most acute lower GI bleeding originates from the colon however 15 to 20 percent of episodes arise from the small intestine and the upper GI tract.

   B. **Elderly patients.** Diverticulosis and angiodysplasia are the most common causes of lower GI bleeding.

   C. **Younger patients.** Hemorrhoids, anal fissures and inflammatory bowel disease are most common causes of lower GI bleeding.

IV. **Diagnosis and management of lower gastrointestinal bleeding**

   A. **Rapid clinical evaluation and resuscitation** should precede diagnostic studies. Intravenous fluids (1 to 2 liters) should be infused over 10- 20 minutes to restore intravascular volume, and blood should be transfused if there is rapid ongoing blood loss or if hypotension or tachycardia are present. Coagulopathy is corrected with fresh frozen plasma, platelets, and cryoprecipitate.

   B. When small amounts of bright red blood are passed per rectum, then lower GI tract can be assumed to be the source. In patients with large volume maroon stools, nasogastric tube aspiration should be performed to exclude massive upper gastrointestinal hemorrhage.

   C. If the nasogastric aspirate contains no blood then anoscopy and sigmoidoscopy should be performed to determine weather a colonic mucosal abnormality (ischemic or infectious colitis) or hemorrhoids might be the cause of bleeding.

   D. **Colonoscopy** in a patient with massive lower GI bleeding is often nondiagnostic, but it can detect ulcerative colitis, antibiotic-associated colitis, or ischemic colon.

   E. **Polyethylene glycol-electrolyte solution** (Colyte or GoLytely) should be administered by means of a nasogastric tube (Four liters of solution is given over a 2-3 hour period), allowing for diagnostic and therapeutic colonoscopy.

V. **Definitive management of lower gastrointestinal bleeding**

   A. **Colonoscopy**

      1. **Colonoscopy** is the procedure of choice for diagnosing colonic causes of GI bleeding. It should be performed after adequate preparation of the bowel. If the bowel cannot be adequately prepared because of persistent, acute bleeding, a bleeding scan or angiography is preferable.

      2. **Endoscopy** may be therapeutic for angiodysplastic lesions, or polyps, which can be coagulated.

      3. If colonoscopy fails to reveal the source of the bleeding, the patient should be observed because, in 80% of cases, bleeding ceases spontaneously.

   B. **Radionuclide scan or bleeding scan.** Technetium- labeled (tagged) red blood cell bleeding scans can detect bleeding sites when bleeding is intermittent. Localization may not he a precise enough to allow segmental colon resection.

C. **Angiography**. Selective mesenteric angiography detects arterial bleeding that occurs at rates of 0.5 mL/per minute or faster. Diverticular bleeding causes pooling of contrast medium within a diverticulum. Bleeding angiodysplastic lesions appear as abnormal vasculature. When active bleeding is seen with diverticular disease or angiodysplasia, selective arterial infusion of vasopressin may be effective.

D. **Surgery**
   1. If bleeding continues and no source can be found, surgical intervention is usually warranted.
   2. Surgical resection may be indicated for patients with recurrent diverticular bleeding, or for patients who have had persistent bleeding from colonic angiodysplasia and have required blood transfusions. Treatment of lower gastrointestinal bleeding involves resection of the involved segments.

VI. **Angiodysplasia**
   A. Angiodysplastic lesions are small vascular tufts that are formed by capillaries, veins and venules, appearing on colonoscopy as red dots or to 2 to 10 mm spider-like lesions. Angiodysplastic lesions developed secondary to chronic colonic distention, and they have a prevalence of 25 percent in elderly patients.
   B. The most common site of bleeding is the right colon. Most patients with angiodysplasia have recurrent minor bleeding; however, massive bleeding may occur.

VII. **Diverticular disease**
   A. Diverticular disease is the most common cause of acute lower gastrointestinal bleeding. Approximately 60-80% of bleeding diverticula are located in the right colon. About 90% of all diverticula are found in the left colon.
   B. Diverticular bleeding tends to be massive, but it stops spontaneously in 80% of patients. The rate of rebleeding is 25%.

VIII. **Colon polyps and colon cancers**
   A. Colonic polyps and colonic cancers rarely cause significant acute lower GI bleeding. Left sided and rectal neoplasms are more likely to cause gross bleeding than right-sided lesions. Right-sided lesions are more likely to cause anemia and occult bleeding.
   B. Diagnosis and treatment of colonic polyps consists of colonoscopic excision or surgical resection.

IX. **Inflammatory bowel disease**
   A. Ulcerative colitis can occasionally cause severe gastrointestinal bleeding associated with the abdominal pain and diarrhea.
   B. Colonoscopy and biopsy is diagnostic, and therapy consists of medical treatment of the underlying disease. Resection is required occasionally.

X. **Ischemic colitis**
   A. Ischemic colitis is seen in elderly patients with known vascular disease. The abdomen pain may be postprandial and associated with bloody diarrhea or rectal bleeding. Severe blood loss is unusual but can occur.
   B. Abdominal films may reveal "thumb-printing" caused by submucosal edema. Colonoscopy reveals a well-demarcated area of hyperemia, edema and mucosal ulcerations. The splenic flexure and descending colon are the most common sites. Most episodes resolve spontaneously, however, vascular bypass or resection may be required.

XI. **Hemorrhoids**
   A. Hemorrhoids rarely cause massive acute blood loss. In patients with portal hypertension, rectal varices should be considered.

B. Diagnosis is by anoscopy and sigmoidoscopy. Treatment consists of high-fiber diets, stool softeners, and/or hemorrhoidectomy.

Acute Pancreatitis

Blanding U. Jones, MD and Russell A. Williams, MD

The incidence of acute pancreatitis ranges from 54 to 238 episodes per 1 million per year. Patients with mild pancreatitis respond well to conservative therapy, but those with severe pancreatitis may have a progressively downhill course to respiratory failure, sepsis, and death (less than 10%).

I. **Etiology**
A. **Alcohol-induced pancreatitis.** Consumption of large quantities of alcohol may cause acute pancreatitis.
B. **Cholelithiasis.** Common bile duct or pancreatic duct obstruction by a stone may cause acute pancreatitis. (90% of all cases of pancreatitis occur secondary to alcohol consumption or cholelithiasis).
C. **Idiopathic pancreatitis.** The cause of pancreatitis cannot be determined in 10 percent of patients.
D. **Hypertriglyceridemia.** Elevation of serum triglycerides (>l,000mg/dL) has been linked with acute pancreatitis.
E. **Pancreatic duct disruption.** In younger patients, a malformation of the pancreatic ducts (eg, pancreatic divisum) with subsequent obstruction is often the cause of pancreatitis. In older patients without an apparent underlying etiology, cancerous lesions of the ampulla of Vater, pancreas or duodenum must be ruled out as possible causes of obstructive pancreatitis.
F. **Iatrogenic pancreatitis.** Radiocontrast studies of the hepatobiliary system (eg, cholangiogram, ERCP) can cause acute pancreatitis in 2-3% of patients undergoing studies.
G. **Trauma.** Blunt or penetrating trauma of any kind to the peri-pancreatic or peri-hepatic regions may induce acute pancreatitis. Extensive surgical manipulation can also induce pancreatitis during laparotomy.

Causes of Acute Pancreatitis	
Alcoholism	Infections
Cholelithiasis	Microlithiasis
Drugs	Pancreas divisum
Hypertriglyceridemia	Trauma
Idiopathic causes	

Medications Associated with Acute Pancreatitis	
Asparaginase (Elspar)	Mercaptopurine (Purinethol)
Azathioprine (Imuran)	Pentamidine
Didanosine (Videx)	Sulfonamides
Estrogens	Tetracyclines
Ethacrynic acid (Edecrin)	Thiazide diuretics
Furosemide (Lasix)	Valproic acid (Depakote)

II. **Pathophysiology.** Acute pancreatitis results when an initiating event causes the extrusion of zymogen granules, from pancreatic acinar cells, into the interstitium of the pancreas. Zymogen particles cause the activation of trypsinogen into trypsin. Trypsin causes auto-digestion of pancreatic tissues.

III. **Clinical presentation**

    A. **Signs and symptoms.** Pancreatitis usually presents with mid-epigastric pain that radiates to the back, associated with nausea and vomiting. The pain is sudden in onset, progressively increases in intensity, and becomes constant. The severity of pain often causes the patient to move continuously in search of a more comfortable position.

    B. **Physical examination**

        1. Patients with acute pancreatitis often appear very ill. Findings that suggest severe pancreatitis include hypotension and tachypnea with decreased basilar breath sounds. Flank ecchymoses (Grey Tuner's Sign) or pedumbilical ecchymoses (Cullen's sign) may be indicative of hemorrhagic pancreatitis.

        2. Abdominal distension and tenderness in the epigastrium are common. Fever and tachycardia are often present. Guarding, rebound tenderness, and hypoactive or absent bowel sounds indicate peritoneal irritation. Deep palpation of abdominal organs should be avoided in the setting of suspected pancreatitis.

IV. **Laboratory testing**

    A. **Leukocytosis.** An elevated WBC with a left shift and elevated hematocrit (indicating hemoconcentration) and hyperglycemia are common. Prerenal azotemia may result from dehydration. Hypoalbuminemia, hypertriglyceridemia, hypocalcemia, hyperbilirubinemia, and mild elevations of transaminases and alkaline phosphatase are common.

    B. **Elevated amylase.** An elevated amylase level often confirms the clinical diagnosis of pancreatitis.

    C. **Elevated lipase.** Lipase measurements are more specific for pancreatitis than amylase levels, but less sensitive. Hyperlipasemia may also occur in patients with renal failure, perforated ulcer disease, bowel infarction and bowel obstruction.

    D. **Abdominal Radiographs** may reveal non-specific findings of pancreatitis, such as "sentinel loops" (dilated loops of small bowel in the vicinity of the pancreas), ileus and, pancreatic calcifications.

    E. **Ultrasonography** demonstrates the entire pancreas in only 20 percent of patients with acute pancreatitis. Its greatest utility is in evaluation of patients with possible gallstone disease.

    F. **Helical high resolution computed tomography** is the imaging modality of choice in acute pancreatitis. CT findings will be normal in 14-29% of patients with mild pancreatitis. Pancreatic necrosis, pseudocysts and abscesses are readily detected by CT.

Selected Conditions Other Than Pancreatitis Associated with Amylase Elevation

Carcinoma of the pancreas	Acute alcoholism
Common bile duct obstruction	Diabetic ketoacidosis
Post-ERCP	Lung cancer
Mesenteric infarction	Ovarian neoplasm
Pancreatic trauma	Renal failure
Perforated viscus	Ruptured ectopic pregnancy
Renal failure	Salivary gland infection
	Macroamylasemia

V. Prognosis. Ranson's criteria is used to determine prognosis in acute pancreatitis. Patients with two or fewer risk factors have a mortality rate of less than 1 percent, those with three or four risk-factors a mortality rate of 16 percent, five or six risk factors, a mortality rate of 40 percent, and seven or eight risk factors, a mortality rate approaching 100 percent.

Ranson's Criteria for Acute Pancreatitis

At admission	During initial 48 hours
1. Age >55 years	1. Hematocrit drop >10%
2. WBC >16,000/mm^3	2. BUN rise >5 mg/dL
3. Blood glucose >200 mg/dL	3. Arterial pO$_2$ <60 mm Hg
4. Serum LDH >350 IU/L	4. Base deficit >4 mEq/L
5. AST >250 U/L	5. Serum calcium <8.0 mg/dL
	6. Estimated fluid sequestration >6 L

VI. Treatment of pancreatitis

   A. Expectant management. Most cases of acute pancreatitis will improve within three to seven days. Management consists of prevention of complications of severe pancreatitis.

   B. NPO and bowel rest. Patients should take nothing by mouth. Total parenteral nutrition should be instituted for those patients fasting for more than five days. A nasogastric tube is warranted if vomiting or ileus.

   C. IV fluid resuscitation. Vigorous intravenous hydration is necessary. A decrease in urine output to less than 30 mL per hour is an indication of inadequate fluid replacement.

   D. Pain control. Morphine is discouraged because it may cause Oddi's sphincter spasm, which may exacerbate the pancreatitis. Meperidine (Demerol), 25-100 mg IV/IM q4-6h, is favored. Ketorolac (Toradol), 60 mg IM/IV, then 15-30 mg IM/IV q6h, is also used.

   E. Antibiotics. Routine use of antibiotics is not recommended in most cases of acute pancreatitis. In cases of infectious pancreatitis, treatment with cefoxitin (1-2 g IV q6h), cefotetan (1-2 g IV q12h), imipenem (1.0 gm IV q6h), or ampicillin/sulbactam (1.5-3.0 g IV q6h) may be appropriate.

   F. Alcohol withdrawal prophylaxis. Alcoholics may require alcohol withdrawal prophylaxis with lorazepam (Ativan) 1-2mg IM/IV q4-6h as needed x 3 days, thiamine 100mg IM/IV qd x 3 days, folic acid 1 mg IM/IV qd x 3 days, multivitamin qd.

G. **Octreotide.** Somatostatin is also a potent inhibitor of pancreatic exocrine secretion. Octreotide is a somatostatin analogue, which has been effective in reducing mortality from bile-induced pancreatitis. Clinical trials, however, have failed to document a significant reduction in mortality

H. **Blood sugar monitoring and insulin administration.** Serum glucose levels should be monitored.

VII. **Complications**
 A. Chronic pancreatitis
 B. Severe hemorrhagic pancreatitis
 C. Pancreatic pseudocysts
 D. Infectious pancreatitis with development of sepsis (occurs in up to 5% of all patients with pancreatitis)
 E. Portal vein thrombosis

Hepatic Encephalopathy

Hepatic encephalopathy develops when ammonia and toxins, which are usually metabolized (detoxified) by the liver, enter into the systemic circulation. Hepatic encephalopathy can be diagnosed in 50-70% of patients with chronic hepatic failure.

I. **Clinical manifestations**
 A. Hepatic encephalopathy manifests as mild changes in personality to altered motor functions and/or level of consciousness.
 B. Most episodes are precipitated by identifiable factors, including gastrointestinal bleeding, excessive protein intake, constipation, excessive diuresis, hypokalemia, hyponatremia or hypernatremia, azotemia, infection, poor compliance with lactulose therapy, sedatives (benzodiazepines, barbiturates, antiemetics), hepatic insult (alcohol, drugs, viral hepatitis), surgery, or hepatocellular carcinoma.
 C. **Hepatic encephalopathy** is a diagnosis of exclusion. Therefore, if a patient with acute or chronic liver failure suddenly develops altered mental status, concomitant problems must be excluded, such as intracranial lesions (hemorrhage, infarct, tumor, abscess), infections (meningitis, encephalitis, sepsis), metabolic encephalopathies (hyperglycemia or hypoglycemia, uremia, electrolyte imbalance), alcohol intoxication or withdrawal, Wernicke's encephalopathy, drug toxicity (sedatives, psychoactive medications), or postictal encephalopathy.
 D. **Physical exam** may reveal hepatosplenomegaly, ascites, jaundice, spider angiomas, gynecomastia, testicular atrophy, and asterixis.
 E. **Computed tomography** may be useful to exclude intracranial abscess or hemorrhage. Laboratory evaluation may include serum ammonia, CBC, electrolyte panel, liver profile, INR/PTT, UA, and blood cultures.

II. **Treatment of hepatic encephalopathy**
 A. **Flumazenil (Romazicon)** may transiently improve the mental state in patients with hepatic encephalopathy. Dosage is 0.2 mg (2 mL) IV over 30 seconds q1min until a total dose of 3 mg; if a partial response occurs, continue 0.5 mg doses until a total of 5 mg. Excessive doses of flumazenil may precipitate seizures.

B. Lactulose is a non-absorbable disaccharide, which decreases the absorption of ammonia into the blood stream. Lactulose can be given orally, through a nasogastric tube, or rectally (less effective). The dosage is 30-45 mL PO q1h x 3 doses, then 15-45 mL PO bid-qid titrate to produce 2-4 soft stools/d. A laxative such as magnesium sulfate and an enema are given before lactulose therapy is started. Lactulose enema (300 mL of lactulose in 700 mL of tap water), 250 mL PR q6h.

C. Neomycin, a poorly absorbed antibiotic, alters intestinal flora and reduces the release of ammonia into the blood (initially 1-2 g orally four times a day). Because chronic neomycin use can cause nephrotoxicity and ototoxicity, neomycin should be used for short periods of time, and the dose should be decreased to 1-2 g/day after achievement of the desired clinical effect. Alternatively, metronidazole can be given at 250 mg orally three times a day alone or with neomycin.

D. Dietary protein is initially withheld, and intravenous glucose is administered to prevent excessive endogenous protein breakdown. As the patient improves, dietary protein can be reinstated at a level of 20 gm per day and then increased gradually to a minimum of 60 gm per day. If adequate oral intake of protein cannot be achieved, therapy with oral or enteral formulas of casein hydrolysates (Ensure) or amino acids (FreAmine) is indicated.

References

Besson I, et al: Sclerotherapy with or without octreotide for acute variceal bleeding, N Eng J Med 333(9): 555-60, 1995.

Adams L; Soulen MC. TIPS: a New Alternative for the Variceal Bleeder. Am J Crit Care 2:196, 1993.

Grate ND: Diagnosis and treatment of gastrointestinal bleeding secondary to protal hypertension. AJG 1997; 92(7): 1081-91

Riordan SM; Williams R: Treatment of hepatic encephalopathy. NEJM 1997; 337(7): 473-79

Haber PS; Perola EC; Wilson JS: Clinical update: management of acute pancreatitis. J of hepatology 1997; 12(3): 189-97

Toxicology

Hans Poggemeyer, MD

Poisoning and Drug Overdose

I. **Management of poisoning and drug overdose**
   A. Stabilize vital signs; maintain airway, breathing and circulation.
   B. Consider intubation if patient has depressed mental status and is at risk for aspiration or respiratory failure.
   C. Establish IV access and administer oxygen.
   D. Draw blood for baseline labs (see below).
   E. If altered mental status is present, administer D50W 50 mL IV push, followed by naloxone (Narcan) 2 mg IV, followed by thiamine 100 mg IV.

II. **Gastrointestinal decontamination**
   A. **Gastric lavage**
      1. Studies have challenged the safety and efficacy of gastric lavage. Lavage retrieves less than 30% of the toxic agent when performed 1 hour after ingestion. Gastric lavage may propel toxins into the duodenum, and accidental placement of the tube into the trachea or mainstem bronchus may occur.
      2. Gastric lavage may be considered if the patient has ingested a potentially life-threatening amount of poison and the procedure can be undertaken within 60 minutes of ingestion.
      3. **Contraindications:** Acid, alkali, or hydrocarbons.
      4. Place the patient in Trendelenburg's position and left lateral decubitus. Insert a large bore (32-40) french Ewald orogastric tube. A smaller NG tube may be used but may be less effective in retrieving large particles.
      5. After tube placement has been confirmed by auscultation, aspirate stomach contents and lavage with 200 cc aliquots of saline or water until clear (up to 2 L). The first 100 cc of fluid should be sent for toxicology analysis.
   B. **Activated charcoal**
      1. Activated charcoal is not effective for alcohols, aliphatic hydrocarbons, caustics, cyanide, elemental metals (boric acid, iron, lithium, lead), or pesticides.
      2. The oral or nasogastric dose is 50 gm mixed with sorbitol. The dose should be repeated at 25-50 gm q4-6h for 24-48 hours if massive ingestion, sustained release products, tricyclic antidepressants, phenothiazines, sertraline (Zoloft), paroxetine (Paxil), carbamazepine, digoxin, phenobarbital, phenytoin, valproate, salicylate, doxepin, or theophylline were ingested.
      3. Give oral cathartic (70% sorbitol) with charcoal.
   C. **Whole bowel irrigation**
      1. Whole bowel irrigation can prevent further absorption in cases of massive ingestion, delayed presentation, or in overdoses of enteric coated or sustained release pills. This treatment may be useful in eliminating objects, such as batteries, or ingested packets of drugs.
      2. Administer GoLytely, or Colyte orally at 1.6-2.0 liter per hour until fecal effluent is clear.

    D. Hemodialysis: Indications include ingestion of phenobarbital, theophylline, chloral hydrate, salicylate, ethanol, lithium, ethylene glycol, isopropyl alcohol, procainamide, and methanol, or severe metabolic acidosis.

    E. Hemoperfusion: May be more effective than hemodialysis **except** for bromides, heavy metals, lithium, and ethylene glycol. Hemoperfusion is effective for disopyramide, phenytoin, barbiturates, theophylline.

Toxicologic Syndromes

I. Characteristics of common toxicologic syndromes

    A. Cholinergic poisoning: Salivation, bradycardia, defecation, lacrimation, emesis, urination, miosis.

    B. Anticholinergic poisoning: Dry skin, flushing, fever, urinary retention, mydriasis, thirst, delirium, conduction delays, tachycardia, ileus.

    C. Sympathomimetic poisoning: Agitation, hypertension, seizure, tachycardia, mydriasis, vasoconstriction.

    D. Narcotic poisoning: Lethargy, hypotension, hypoventilation, miosis, coma, ileus.

    E. Withdrawal syndrome: Diarrhea, lacrimation, mydriasis, cramps, tachycardia, hallucination.

    F. Salicylate poisoning: Fever, respiratory alkalosis, or mixed acid-base disturbance, hyperpnea, hypokalemia, tinnitus.

    G. Causes of toxic seizures: Amoxapine, anticholinergics, camphor, carbon monoxide, cocaine, ergotamine, isoniazid, lead, lindane, lithium, LSD, parathion, phencyclidine, phenothiazines, propoxyphene propranolol, strychnine, theophylline, tricyclic antidepressants, normeperidine (metabolite of meperidine), thiocyanate.

    H. Causes of toxic cardiac arrhythmias: Arsenic, beta-blockers, chloral hydrate, chloroquine, clonidine, calcium channel blockers, cocaine, cyanide, carbon monoxide, digitalis, ethanol, phenol, phenothiazine, tricyclics.

    I. Extrapyramidal syndromes: Dysphagia, dysphonia, trismus, rigidity, torticollis, laryngospasm.

Acetaminophen Overdose

I. Clinical features

    A. Acute lethal dose = 13-25 g. Acetaminophen is partly metabolized to N-acetyl-p-benzoquinonimine which is conjugated by glutathione. Hepatic glutathione stores can be depleted in acetaminophen overdose, leading to centrilobular hepatic necrosis.

    B. Liver failure occurs 3 days after ingestion if untreated. Liver failure presents with right upper quadrant pain, elevated liver function tests, coagulopathy, hypoglycemia, renal failure and encephalopathy.

II. Treatment

    A. Gastrointestinal decontamination should consist of gastric lavage followed by activated charcoal. Residual charcoal should be removed with saline lavage prior to giving N-acetyl-cysteine (NAC).

B. Check acetaminophen level 4 hours after ingestion. A nomogram should be used to determine if treatment is necessary (see next page). Start treatment if level is above the nontoxic range or if the level is potentially toxic but the time of ingestion is unknown.

C. Therapy must start no later than 8-12 hours after ingestion. Treatment after 16-24 hours of non-sustained release formulation is significantly less effective, but should still be accomplished.

D. Oral N-acetyl-cysteine (Mucomyst): 140 mg/kg PO followed by 70 mg/kg PO q4h x 17 doses (total 1330 mg/kg over 72 h). Repeat loading dose if emesis occurs Complete all doses even after acetaminophen level falls below critical value.

E. Hemodialysis and hemoperfusion are somewhat effective, but should not take the place of NAC treatment.

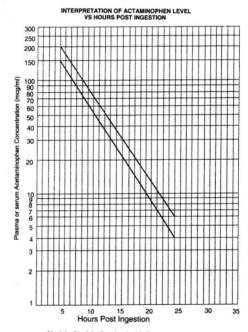

INTERPRETATION OF ACTAMINOPHEN LEVEL
VS HOURS POST INGESTION

No risk of toxicity if under double lines.
Probable risk if above top line.
Possible risk if between double lines.
Outcome is best if treatment is initiated within 12 hours of ingestion.
Graph applies to non-sustained release formulations only .

Cocaine Overdose

I. Clinical evaluation

- **A.** Cocaine can be used intravenously, smoked, ingested, or inhaled nasally. Street cocaine often is cut with other substances including amphetamines, LSD, PCP, heroin, strychnine, lidocaine, talc, and quinine.
- **B.** One-third of fatalities occur within 1 hour, with another third occurring 6-24 hours later.
- **C.** Persons may transport cocaine by swallowing wrapped packets, and some users may hastily swallow packets of cocaine to avoid arrest.

II. Clinical features

- **A. CNS:** Sympathetic stimulation, agitation, seizures, tremor, headache, subarachnoid hemorrhage, ischemic cerebral stoke, psychosis, hallucinations, fever, mydriasis, formication (sensation of insects crawling on skin).
- **B. Cardiovascular:** Atrial and ventricular arrhythmias, myocardial infarction, hypertension, hypotension, myocarditis, aortic rupture, cardiomyopathy.
- **C. Pulmonary:** Noncardiogenic pulmonary edema, pneumomediastinum, alveolar hemorrhage, hypersensitivity pneumonitis, bronchiolitis obliterans.
- **D. Other:** Rhabdomyolysis, mesenteric ischemia, hepatitis.

III. Treatment

- **A.** Treatment consists of supportive care because no antidote exists. GI decontamination, including repeated activated charcoal, whole bowel irrigation and endoscopic evaluation is provided if oral ingestion is suspected.
- **B.** Hyperadrenergic symptoms should be treated with benzodiazepines, such as lorazepam.
- **C. Seizures:** Treat with lorazepam, phenytoin, or phenobarbital.
- **D. Arrhythmias**
  1. Treat hyperadrenergic state and supraventricular tachycardia with lorazepam and propranolol.
  2. Ventricular arrhythmias are treated with lidocaine or propranolol.
- **E. Hypertension**
  1. Use lorazepam first for tachycardia and hypertension.
  2. If no response, use labetalol because it has alpha and beta blocking effects.
  3. If hypertension remains severe, administer sodium nitroprusside or esmolol drip.
- **F. Myocardial ischemia and infarction:** Treat with thrombolysis, heparin, aspirin, beta-blockers, nitroglycerin. Control hypertension and exclude CNS bleeding before using thrombolytic therapy.

Cyclic Antidepressant Overdose

I. Clinical features

A. Antidepressants have prolonged body clearance rates, and cannot be removal by forced diuresis, hemodialysis, and hemoperfusion. Delayed absorption is common because of decreased GI motility from anticholinergic effects. Cyclic antidepressants undergo extensive enterohepatic recirculation.

B. **CNS:** Lethargy, coma, hallucinations, seizures, myoclonic jerks.

C. **Anticholinergic crises:** Blurred vision, dilated pupils, urinary retention, dry mouth, ileus, hyperthermia.

D. **Cardiac:** Hypotension, ventricular tachyarrhythmias, sinus tachycardia.

E. **ECG:** Sinus tachycardia, right bundle branch block, right axis deviation, increased PR and QT interval, QRS >100 msec, or right axis deviation. Prolongation of the QRS width is a more reliable predictor of CNS and cardiac toxicity than the serum level.

II. Treatment

A. **Gastrointestinal decontamination and systemic drug removal**

1. Magnesium citrate 300 mL via nasogastric tube x 1 dose.

2. Activated charcoal premixed with sorbitol 50 gm via nasogastric tube q4-6h around-the-clock until the serum level decreases to therapeutic range. Maintain the head-of-bed at a 30-45 degree angle to prevent aspiration.

3. **Cardiac toxicity**

   a. Alkalinization is a cardioprotective measure and it has no influence on drug elimination. The goal of treatment is to achieve an arterial pH of 7.50-7.55. If mechanical ventilation is necessary, hyperventilate to maintain desired pH.

   b. Administer sodium bicarbonate 50-100 mEq (1-2 amps or 1-2 mEq/kg) IV over 5-10 min. Followed by infusion of sodium bicarbonate, 2 amps in 1 liter of D5W at 100-150 cc/h. Adjust IV rate to maintain desired pH.

4. **Seizures**

   a. Administer lorazepam or diazepam IV followed by phenytoin.

   b. Physostigmine, 1-2 mg slow IV over 3-4 min, is necessary if seizures continue.

Digoxin Overdose

I. Clinical features

A. The therapeutic window of digoxin is 0.8-2.0 ng/mL. Drugs that increase digoxin levels include verapamil, quinidine, amiodarone, flecainide, erythromycin, and tetracycline. Hypokalemia, hypomagnesemia and hypercalcemia enhance digoxin toxicity.

B. **CNS:** Confusion, lethargy; yellow-green visual halo.

C. **Cardiac:** Common dysrhythmias include ventricular tachycardia or fibrillation; variable atrioventricular block, atrioventricular dissociation; sinus bradycardia, junctional tachycardia, premature ventricular contractions.

D. **GI:** Nausea, vomiting.

    E. Metabolic: Hypokalemia enhances the toxic effects of digoxin on the myocardial tissue and may be present in patients on diuretics.

II. Treatment

    A. Gastrointestinal decontamination: Gastric lavage, followed by repeated doses of activated charcoal, is effective; hemodialysis is ineffective.

    B. Treat bradycardia with atropine, isoproterenol, and cardiac pacing.

    C. Treat ventricular arrhythmias with lidocaine or phenytoin. Avoid procainamide and quinidine because they are proarrhythmic and slow AV conduction.

    D. Electrical DC cardioversion may be dangerous in severe toxicity. Hypomagnesemia and hypokalemia should be corrected.

    E. Digibind (Digoxin - specific Fab antibody fragment)

        1. Indication: Life-threatening arrhythmias refractory to conventional therapy.

        2. Dosage of Digoxin immune Fab:

$$\text{(number of 40 mg vials)} = \frac{\text{Digoxin level (ng/mL) x body weight (kg)}}{100}$$

        3. Dissolve the digoxin immune Fab in 100-150 mL of NS and infuse IV over 15-30 minutes. A 0.22 micron in-line filter should be used during infusion.

        4. Hypokalemia, heart failure, and anaphylaxis may occur. The complex is renally excreted; after administration, serum digoxin levels may be artificially high because both free and bound digoxin is measured.

Ethylene Glycol Ingestion

I. Clinical features

    A. Ethylene glycol is found in antifreeze, detergents, and polishes.

    B. Toxicity: Half-life 3-5 hours; the half-life increases to 17 hours if coingested with alcohol. The minimal lethal dose is 1.0-1.5 cc/kg, and the lethal blood level is 200 mg/dL.

    C. Anion gap metabolic acidosis and severe osmolar gap is often present. CNS depression and cranial nerve dysfunction (facial and vestibulocochlear palsies) are common.

    D. GI symptoms such as flank pain. Oxalate crystals may be seen in the urine sediment. Other findings may include hypocalcemia (due to calcium oxalate formation); tetany, seizures, and prolonged QT.

II. Treatment

    A. Fomepizole (Antizol) loading dose 15 mg/kg IV; then 10 mg/kg IV q12h x 4, then 15 mg/kg IV q12h until ethylene glycol level is <20 mg/dL.

    B. Pyridoxine 100 mg IV qid x 2 days and thiamine 100 mg IV qid x 2 days.

    C. If definitive therapy is not immediately available, 3-4 ounces of whiskey (or equivalent) may be given orally.

    D. Hemodialysis indications: Severe refractory metabolic acidosis, crystalluria, serum ethylene glycol level >50 mg/dL; keep glycol level <10 mg/dL.

Gamma-hydroxybutyrate Ingestion

I. **Clinical features**
   A. Gamma-hydroxybutyrate (GHB) was used as an anesthetic agent but was banned because of the occurrence of seizures. Gamma-hydroxybutyrate is now an abused substance at dance clubs because of the euphoric effects of the drug. It is also abused by body builders because of a mistaken belief that it has anabolic properties. Gamma-hydroxybutyrate is a clear, odorless, oily, salty liquid. It is rapidly absorbed within 20-40 minutes of ingestion and metabolized in the liver. The half-life of GHB is 20-30 min.
   B. Gamma-hydroxybutyrate is not routinely included on toxicological screens, but it can be detected in the blood and urine by gas chromatography within 12 hours of ingestion. Gamma hydroxybutyrate may cause respiratory depression, coma, seizures, and severe agitation. Cardiac effects include hypotension, cardiac arrest, and severe vomiting.

II. **Treatment**
   A. Gastric lavage is not indicated due to rapid absorption of GHB.
   B. Immediate care consists of support of ventilation and circulation. Agitation should be treated with benzodiazepines, haloperidol, or propofol. Seizures should be treated with lorazepam, phenytoin, or valproic acid.

Iron Overdose

I. **Clinical features**
   A. Toxicity is caused by free radical organ damage to the GI mucosa, liver, kidney, heart, and lungs. The cause of death is usually shock and liver failure.

Toxic dosages and serum levels	
Nontoxic	<10-20 mg/kg of elemental iron (0-100 mcg/dL)
Toxic	>20 mg/kg of elemental iron (350-1000 mcg/dL)
Lethal	>180-300 mg/kg of elemental iron (>1000 mcg/dL)

   B. **Two hours after ingestion:** Severe hemorrhagic gastritis; vomiting, diarrhea, lethargy, tachycardia, and hypotension.
   C. **Twelve hours after ingestion:** Improvement and stabilization.
   D. **12-48 hours after ingestion:** GI bleeding, coma, seizures, pulmonary edema, circulatory collapse, hepatic and renal failure, coagulopathy, hypoglycemia, and severe metabolic acidosis.

II. **Treatment**
   A. Administer deferoxamine if iron levels reach toxic values. Deferoxamine 100 mg binds 9 mg of free elemental iron. The deferoxamine dosage is 10-15 mg/kg/hr IV infusion.

    B. Treat until 24 hours after vin rose colored urine clears. Serum iron levels during chelation are not accurate. Deferoxamine can cause hypotension, allergic reactions such as pruritus, urticarial wheals, rash, anaphylaxis, tachycardia, fever, and leg cramps.

    C. Gastrointestinal decontamination

        1. Charcoal is not effective in absorbing elemental iron. Abdominal x-rays should be evaluated for remaining iron tablets. Consider whole bowel lavage if iron pills are past the stomach and cannot be removed by gastric lavage (see page 105).

        2. Hemodialysis is indicated for severe toxicity.

Isopropyl Alcohol Ingestion

I. Clinical features

    A. Isopropyl alcohol is found in rubbing alcohol, solvents, and antifreeze.

    B. Toxicity: Lethal dose: 3-4 g/kg

        1. Lethal blood level: 400 mg/dL

        2. Half-life = 3 hours

    C. Metabolism: Isopropyl alcohol is metabolized to acetone. Toxicity is characterized by an anion gap metabolic acidosis with high serum ketone level; mild osmolar gap; mildly elevated glucose.

    D. CNS depression, headache, nystagmus; cardiovascular depression, abdominal pain and vomiting, and pulmonary edema may occur.

II. Treatment

    A. Treatment consists of supportive care. No antidote is available; ethanol is not indicated.

    B. Hemodialysis: Indications: refractory hypotension, coma, potentially lethal blood levels.

Lithium Overdose

I. Clinical features

    A. Lithium has a narrow therapeutic window of 0.8-1.2 mEq/L.

    B. Drugs that will increase lithium level include NSAIDs, phenothiazines, thiazide and loop diuretics (by causing hyponatremia).

    C. Toxicity

        1.5-3.0 mEq/L = moderate toxicity

        3.0-4.0 mEq/L = severe toxicity

    D. Toxicity in chronic lithium users occurs at much lower serum levels than with acute ingestions.

    E. Common manifestations include seizures, encephalopathy, hyperreflexia, tremor, nausea, vomiting, diarrhea, hypotension. Nephrogenic diabetes insipidus and hypothyroidism may also occur. Conduction block and dysrhythmias are rare, but reversible T-wave depression may occur.

II. Treatment

    A. Correct hyponatremia with aggressive normal saline hydration. Follow lithium levels until <1.0 mEq/L.

    B. Forced solute diuresis: Hydrate with normal saline infusion to maintain urine output at 2-4 cc/kg/hr; use furosemide (Lasix) 40-80 mg IV doses as needed.

C. **GI decontamination**
1. Administer gastric lavage. Activated charcoal is ineffective. Whole bowel irrigation may be useful.
2. **Indications for hemodialysis:** Level >4 mEq/L; CNS or cardiovascular impairment with level of 2.5-4.0 mEq/L.

Methanol Ingestion

I. **Clinical features**
   A. **Methanol** is found in antifreeze, Sterno, cleaners, and paints.
   B. **Toxicity**
   1. 10 cc causes blindness
   2. Minimal lethal dose = 1-5 g/kg
   3. Lethal blood level = 80 mg/dL
   4. Symptomatic in 40 minutes to 72 hours.
   C. **Signs and Symptoms**
   1. Severe osmolar and anion gap metabolic acidosis.
   2. Visual changes occur because of optic nerve toxicity, leading to blindness.
   3. Nausea, vomiting, abdominal pain, pancreatitis, and altered mental status.
II. **Treatment**
   A. Ethanol 10% is infuse in D5W as 7.5 cc/kg load then 1.4 cc/kg/h drip to keep blood alcohol level between 100-150 mg/dL. Continue therapy until the methanol level is below 20-25 mg/dL.
   B. Give folate 50 mg IV q4h to enhance formic acid metabolism.
   C. Correct acidosis and electrolyte imbalances.
   D. **Hemodialysis:** Indications: peak methanol level >50 mg/dL; formic acid level >20 mg/dL; severe metabolic acidosis; acute renal failure; any visual compromise.

Salicylate Overdose

I. **Clinical features**
   A. **Toxicity**
   150-300 mg/kg - mild toxicity
   300-500 mg/kg - moderate toxicity
   >500 mg/kg - severe toxicity
   B. Chronic use can cause toxicity at much lower levels (ie, 25 mg/dL) than occurs with acute use.
   C. **Acid/Base Abnormalities:** Patients present initially with a respiratory alkalosis because of central hyperventilation. Later an anion gap metabolic acidosis occurs.
   D. **CNS:** Tinnitus, lethargy, irritability, seizures, coma, cerebral edema.
   E. **GI:** Nausea, vomiting, liver failure, GI bleeding.
   F. **Cardiac:** Hypotension, sinus tachycardia, AV block, wide complex tachycardia.
   G. **Pulmonary:** Non-cardiogenic pulmonary edema, adult respiratory distress syndrome.

H. **Metabolic:** Renal failure; coagulopathy because of decreased factor VII; hyperthermia because of uncoupled oxidative phosphorylation. Hypoglycemia may occur in children, but it is rare in adults.

II. **Treatment**
   A. Provide supportive care and GI decontamination. Aspirin may form concretions or drug bezoars, and ingestion of enteric coated preparations may lead to delayed toxicity.
   B. Multiple dose activated charcoal, whole bowel irrigation, and serial salicylate levels are indicated. Hypotension should be treated vigorously with fluids. Abnormalities should be corrected, especially hypokalemia. Urine output should be maintained at 200 cc/h or more. Metabolic acidosis should be treated with bicarbonate 50-100 mEq (1-2 amps) IVP.
   C. Renal clearance is increased by alkalinization of urine with a bicarbonate infusion (2-3 amps in 1 liter of D5W IV at 150-200 mL/h), keeping the urine pH at 7.5-8.5.
   D. **Hemodialysis** is indicated for seizures, cardiac or renal failure, intractable acidosis, acute salicylate level >120 mg/dL or chronic level >50 mg/dL (therapeutic level 15-25 mg/dL).

Theophylline Toxicity

I. **Clinical features**
   A. Drug interactions can increase serum theophylline level, including quinolone and macrolide antibiotics, propranolol, cimetidine, and oral contraceptives. Liver disease or heart failure will decrease clearance.
   B. **Serum toxicity levels**
      20-40 mg/dL - mild
      40-70 mg/dL - moderate
      >70 mg/dL - life threatening
   C. Toxicity in chronic users occurs at lower serum levels than with short-term users. Seizures and arrhythmias can occur at therapeutic or minimally supra-therapeutic levels.
   D. **CNS:** Hyperventilation, agitation, and tonic-clonic seizures.
   E. **Cardiac:** Sinus tachycardia, multi-focal atrial tachycardia, supraventricular tachycardia, ventricular tachycardia and fibrillation, premature ventricular contractions, hypotension or hypertension.
   F. **Gastrointestinal:** Vomiting, diarrhea, hematemesis.
   G. **Musculoskeletal:** Tremor, myoclonic jerks
   H. **Metabolic:** Hypokalemia, hypomagnesemia, hypophosphatemia, hyper-glycemia, and hypercalcemia.

II. **Treatment**
   A. **Gastrointestinal decontamination and systemic drug removal**
      1. Activated charcoal premixed with sorbitol, 50 gm PO or via nasogastric tube q4h around-the-clock until theophylline level is less than 20 mcg/mL. Maintain head-of-bed at 30 degrees to prevent charcoal aspiration.
      2. Hemodialysis is as effective as repeated oral doses of activated charcoal and should be used when charcoal hemoperfusion is not feasible.

3. **Indications for charcoal hemoperfusion:** Coma, seizures, hemodynamic instability, theophylline level >60 mcg/mL; rebound in serum levels may occur after discontinuation of hemoperfusion.
4. **Seizures** are generally refractory to anticonvulsants. High doses of lorazepam, diazepam or phenobarbital should be used; phenytoin is less effective.
5. **Treatment of hypotension**
   a. Normal saline fluid bolus.
   b. Norepinephrine 8-12 mcg/min IV infusion or
   c. Phenylephrine 20-200 mcg/min IV infusion.
6. **Treatment of ventricular arrhythmias**
   a. Amiodarone 150-300 mg IV over 10 min, then 1 mg/min x 6 hours, followed by 0.5 mg/min IV infusion. Lidocaine should be avoided because it has epileptogenic properties.
   b. Esmolol (Brevibloc) 500 mcg/kg/min loading dose, then 50-300 mcg/kg/min continuous IV drip.

Warfarin (Coumadin) Overdose

I. **Clinical management**
   A. **Elimination measures:** Gastric lavage and activated charcoal if recent oral ingestion of warfarin (Coumadin).
   B. **Reversal of coumadin anticoagulation:** Coagulopathy should be corrected rapidly or slowly depending on the following factors: 1) Intensity of hypocoagulability, 2) severity or risk of bleeding, 3) need for reinstitution of anticoagulation.
   C. **Emergent reversal**
      1. **Fresh frozen plasma:** Replace vitamin K dependent factors with FFP 2-4 units; repeat in 4 hours if prothrombin time remains prolonged.
      2. Vitamin K, 25 mg in 50 cc NS, to infuse no faster than 1 mg/min; risk of anaphylactoid reactions and shock; slow infusion minimizes risk.
   D. **Reversal over 24-48 Hours:** Vitamin K 10-25 mg subcutaneously. Full reversal of anticoagulation will result in resistance to further Coumadin therapy for several days.
   E. **Partial correction:** Lower dose vitamin K (0.5-1.0 mg) will lower prothrombin time without interfering with reinitiation of Coumadin.

References

Craig K. Gomez H, et al: Severe Gamma-Hydroxybutyrate Withdrawal: A case report and literature review. J of Emergency Medicine, 2000; 18:65-70.

The American Academy of Clinical Toxicology and the European Association of Poison Control Centers and Clinical Toxicologists position statement on gut decontamination in acute poisoning. J Toxicol-Clin Toxicol 1997; 35:695-762.

Kelly RA, Smith TW: Recognition and management of digitalis toxicity. The American Journal of Cardiology,69:108G, 1992

Markenson D, Greenberg MD: Cyclic Antidepressant overdose: mechanism to management. Emergency Medicine, 25:49, 1993.

Spiller HA, Kreuzelok EP, Grand GA, et al.: A prospective evaluation of the effect of activated charcoal before oral n-acetylcysteine in acetaminophen overdose. Annals of Emergency Medicine, 23:519-523, 1994.

Neurologic Disorders

Hans Poggemeyer, MD

Ischemic Stroke

Ischemic stroke is the third leading cause of death in the United States and the most common cause of neurologic disability in adults. Approximately 85 percent of strokes are ischemic in nature.

I. **Clinical evaluation of the stroke patient**
   A. A rapid evaluation should determine the time when symptoms started. Other diseases that may mimic a stroke, such as seizure disorders, metabolic abnormalities, hypoglycemia, complex migraine, dysrhythmia or syncope, infection, should be excluded.
   B. Markers of vascular disease such as diabetes, angina pectoris and intermittent claudication, are suggestive of ischemic stroke. A history of atrial fibrillation or MI suggests a cardiac embolic stroke.

II. **Physical examination**
   A. Assessment should determine whether the patient's condition is acutely deteriorating or relatively stable. Airway and circulatory stabilization take precedence over diagnostic and therapeutic interventions.
   B. **Neurologic exam.** Evaluation should include the level of consciousness, orientation; ability to speak and understand language; cranial nerve function, especially eye movements, pupil reflexes and facial paresis; neglect, gaze preference, arm and leg strength, sensation, and walking ability.
   C. A semiconscious or unconscious patient probably has a hemorrhage. A patient with an ischemic stroke may be drowsy but is unlikely to lose consciousness unless the infarcted area is large.

III. **CT scanning and diagnostic studies**
   A. All patients with signs of stroke should undergo a noncontrast head CT to screen for bleeding and to rule out expanding lesions, such as subdural hematomas, or epidural hematomas.
   B. CT scanning usually does not show signs of acute ischemia. Within 3 hours of onset, the sensitivity is 30 %, within 24 hours 60%, and 100% at 7 days. Early CT changes include effacement of sulci or ventricles, blurring of the basal ganglia, mass effect, and loss of the normal gray-white junction in the insula.
   C. A complete blood count including platelets, international normalized ratio, activated partial thromboplastin time, serum electrolytes, and a rapid blood glucose should be obtained. ECG, and chest x-ray should be ordered. Arterial blood gas and lumbar puncture should be obtained when indicated.

IV. **Management of ischemic stroke**
   A. **Tissue plasminogen activator (t-PA, Activase).** Use of t-PA within 3 hours of onset of stroke results in complete or near-complete neurological recovery in one-third more patients, compared to placebo, at three and 12 months. The incidence of brain hemorrhage is 10 times higher with t-PA (6.4% vs 0.6% placebo) and occurs predominantly in those

patients with gross neurological deficit, and in the presence of cerebral edema or mass.

B. The CT scan must document the absence of intracranial bleeding before treatment.

Criteria for Thrombolysis of Patients with Acute Ischemic Stroke Using Tissue Plasminogen Activator

Inclusion criteria
Age greater than 18 years
Clinical diagnosis of ischemic stroke, with onset of symptoms within three hours of initiation of treatment
Noncontrast CT scan with no evidence of hemorrhage

Exclusion criteria
History
Stroke or head trauma in previous three months
History of intracranial hemorrhage that may increase risk of recurrent hemorrhage
Major surgery or other serious trauma in previous 14 days
Gastrointestinal or genitourinary bleeding in previous 21 days
Arterial puncture in previous seven days
Pregnant or lactating patient
Clinical findings
Rapidly improving stroke symptoms
Seizure at onset of stroke
Symptoms suggestive of subarachnoid hemorrhage, even if CT scan is normal
Persistent systolic pressure greater than 185 mm Hg or diastolic pressure greater than 110 mm Hg, or patient is requiring aggressive therapy to control blood pressure
Clinical presentation consistent with acute myocardial infarction or postmyocardial infarction pericarditis requires cardiologic evaluation before treatment
Imaging results
CT scan with evidence of hemorrhage
CT scan with evidence of hypodensity and/or effacement of cerebral sulci in more than one-third of middle cerebral artery territory
Laboratory findings
Glucose level less than 50 mg per dL or greater than 400 mg per dL
Platelet count less than 100,000 per mm^3
Warfarin therapy with an international normalized ratio ≥ 1.7
Patient has received heparin within 48 hours, and partial thromboplastin time is increased

Antiplatelet Agents for Prevention of Ischemic Stoke

- Enteric-coated aspirin (Ecotrin) 325 mg PO qd
- Clopidogrel (Plavix) 75 mg PO qd
- Extended-release aspirin 25 mg with dipyridamole 200 mg (Aggrenox) one tab PO qd

  C. **Antiplatelet agents** minimally reduce in the risk of death or disability by about one case per 100 patients. Aspirin, clopidogrel (Plavix), or a combination of low-dose aspirin plus extended-release dipyridamole (Aggrenox) should be initiated after a repeat CT scan (24 hours after t-PA) has excluded hemorrhage due to thrombolysis.

  D. **Antithrombotic therapy.** Heparin has no proven benefit in the treatment of ischemic stroke. In cases of cardioembolic stroke or carotid stenosis, heparin may be initiated 24 hours after t-PA, providing a repeat CT scan at that time shows no hemorrhage. Heparin should be gradually transitioned to warfarin for long-term treatment.

  E. **Cytoprotective agents.** These agents increase the tolerance of neurons to ischemia. Large trials evaluating citicoline, clomethiazole and glycine antagonist should be completed soon.

Initial Management of Acute Stroke

Determine whether stroke is ischemic or hemorrhagic by computed tomography

Consider administration of t-PA if less than three hours from stroke onset

General management:
- Blood pressure (avoid hypotension)
- Assure adequate oxygenation
- Administer intravenous glucose
- Take dysphagia/aspiration precautions
- Consider prophylaxis for venous thrombosis if the patient is unable to walk
- Suppress fever, if present
- Assess stroke mechanism (eg, atrial fibrillation, hypertension)
- Consider aspirin or clopidogrel (Plavix) therapy if ischemic stroke and no contraindications (begin 24 hours after t-PA).

  F. **Thrombolytic therapy.** The dose of t-PA for acute ischemic stroke is 0.9 mg/kg with a maximum dose of 90 mg. Ten percent of the dose is given as a bolus dose, and the remainder is given over 60 minutes. No heparin or anti-platelet agents (aspirin) should be administered until 24 hours after initiation of t-PA treatment and a scan 24 hours after the stroke CT has ruled out intracranial hemorrhage.

  G. **Blood pressure management in thrombolytic therapy**
    1. Arterial blood pressure should be kept just below 185 mm Hg during the first 24 hours.
    2. Severe hypertension should be controlled with labetalol, administered at an initial dose of 10 mg IV over 1-2 minutes. The dose may be repeated or doubled every 10-20 minutes if needed, or an IV infusion

of 2 mg/min may be initiated. If the response is unsatisfactory, then an infusion of sodium nitroprusside starting at an initial dose of 0.1 mcg/kg/min is recommended.

Elevated Intracranial Pressure

Cerebrospinal fluid (CSF) pressure in excess of 250 mm CSF is usually a manifestation of serious neurologic disease. Intracranial hypertension is most often associated with rapidly expanding mass lesions, CSF outflow obstruction, or cerebral venous congestion.

I. **Clinical evaluation**
   A. Increased intracranial pressure may manifest as headache caused by traction on pain-sensitive cerebral blood vessels or dura mater.
   B. Papilledema is the most reliable sign of ICP, although it fails to develop in many patients with increased ICP. Retinal venous pulsations, when present, imply that CSF pressure is normal or not significantly elevated. Patients with increased ICP often complain of worsening headache, in the morning.

Causes of Increased Intracranial Pressure

Diffuse cerebral edema	Space-occupying lesions
Meningitis	Intracerebral hemorrhage
Encephalitis	Epidural hemorrhage
Hepatic encephalopathy	Subdural hemorrhage
Reye's syndrome	Tumor
Acute liver failure	Abscess
Electrolyte shifts	**Hydrocephalus**
Dialysis	Subarachnoid hemorrhage
Hypertensive encephalopathy	Meningitis
Posthypoxic brain injury	Aqueductal stenosis
Lead encephalopathy	Idiopathic
Uncompensated hypercarbia	**Miscellaneous**
Head trauma	Pseudotumor cerebri
Diffuse axonal injury	Craniosynostosis
	Venous sinus thrombosis

II. **Intracranial Pressure Monitoring**
   A. Clinical signs of elevated ICP, such as the Cushing response (systemic hypertension, bradycardia, and irregular respirations), are usually a late findings and may never even occur; therefore, ICP should be directly measured with an invasive device.
   B. Normal intracranial pressures range from approximately 10-20 cm H_2O (or about 5 to 15 mm Hg). Ventricular catheterization involves insertion of a sterile catheter into the lateral ventricle.

Treatment of Elevated Intracranial Pressure			
Treatment	**Dose**	**Advantages**	**Limitations**
Hypocarbia by hyperventilation	pCO_2 25 to 33 mm Hg respiratory rate of 10 to 16/min	Immediate onset, well tolerated	Hypotension, barotrauma, duration usually hours or less
Osmotic	Mannitol 0.5 to 1 g/kg IV push	Rapid onset, titratable, predictable	Hypotension, hypokalemia, duration hours or days
Barbiturates	Pentobarbital 25 mg/kg slow IV infusion over 3-4 hours	Mutes BP and respiratory fluctuations	Hypotension, fixed pupils (small), duration days
Hemicraniectomy	Timing critical	Large sustained ICP reduction	Surgical risk, tissue herniation through wound

III. Treatment of increased intracranial pressure

- **A. Positioning** the patient in an upright position with the head of the bed at 30 degrees will lower ICP.
- **B. Hyperventilation** is the most rapid and effective means of lowering ICP, but the effects are short lived because the body quickly compensates. The pCO_2 should be maintained between 25-33 mm Hg
- **C. Mannitol** can quickly lower ICP, although the effect is not long lasting and may lead to dehydration or electrolyte imbalance. Dosage is 0.5-1 gm/kg (37.5-50 gm) IV q6h; keep osmolarity <315; do not give for more than 48h.
- **D. Corticosteroids** are best used to treat increased ICP in the setting of vasogenic edema caused by brain tumors or abscesses; however, these agents have little value in the setting of stroke or head trauma. Dosage is dexamethasone (Decadron) 10 mg IV or IM, followed by 4-6 mg IV, IM or PO q6h.
- **E. Barbiturate coma** is used for medically intractable ICP elevation when other medical therapies have failed. There is a reduction in ICP by decreasing cerebral metabolism. The pentobarbital loading dose is 25 mg/kg body weight over 3-4 hours, followed by 2-3 mg/kg/hr IV infusion. Blood levels are periodically checked and adjusted to 30-40 mg/dL. Patients require mechanical ventilation, intracranial pressure monitoring, and continuous electroencephalographic monitoring.
- **F. Management of blood pressure.** Beta-blockers or mixed beta and alpha blockers provide the best antihypertensive effects without causing significant cerebral vasodilatation that can lead to elevated ICP.

Status Epilepticus

Status epilepticus (SE) is defined as a continuous seizures lasting at least 5 minutes, or 2 or more discrete seizures between which there is incomplete recovery of consciousness. Simple seizures are characterized by focal motor or sensory phenomena, with full preservation of consciousness. Generalized seizures include generalized tonic-clonic seizures. Complex seizures are diagnosed when an alteration in consciousness has occurred.

I. Diagnostic evaluation
A. Laboratory evaluation
1. **CBC, blood glucose level, serum electrolytes** (sodium, magnesium, calcium), anticonvulsant drug levels, and urinalysis.
2. **Lumbar puncture** is necessary if meningitis or subarachnoid hemorrhage is suspected.
3. **Toxicologic screening** is indicated in specific situations.
B. CT scan is indicated if tumor, abscess, subarachnoid hemorrhage, or trauma is suspected, or if the patient has no prior history of seizures.
C. Electroencephalogram. An immediate EEG may be required if the patient fails to awaken promptly after the seizure.

Etiology of Status Epilepticus

Status epilepticus in a patient with a history of seizure disorder
- Noncompliance with prescribed medical regimen
- Withdrawal seizures from anticonvulsants
- Breakthrough seizures

New onset seizure disorder presenting with status epilepticus

Status epilepticus secondary to medical, toxicologic, or structural symptoms
- Anoxic brain injury
- Stroke syndromes
- Subarachnoid hemorrhage
- Intracranial tumor
- Trauma
- Theophylline, cocaine, amphetamine or isoniazid overdose; alcohol withdrawal, gamma hydroxybutyrate
- Hyponatremia, hypernatremia, hypercalcemia, hypomagnesemia, hepatic encephalopathy
- Meningitis, brain abscess, encephalitis, CNS cysticercosis or toxoplasmosis

---

II. Management of generalized convulsive status epilepticus (GCSE)
A. A history should be obtained, and a brief physical examination performed. **Initial stabilization** consists of airway management, 100% oxygen by mask, rapid glucose testing, intravenous access, and cardiac and hemodynamic monitoring.

B. Initial pharmacologic therapy

1. Thiamine 100 mg IV push and dextrose 50% water (D5W) 50 mL IV push.
2. Lorazepam (Ativan) 0.1 mg/kg IV at 2 mg/min. The same dose may be repeated once. Lorazepam may be given IM if the IV route is unavailable.
3. **Phenytoin** may be used when benzodiazepines are not effective. The loading dose of phenytoin is 20 mg/kg IV, followed by 4-5 mg/kg/day (100 mg IV q8h or 200 mg IV q12h); maximum rate for each dose is 50 mg/min in normal saline only. An additional loading dose of phenytoin 10 mg/kg may be given if necessary.
4. **Fosphenytoin (Cerebyx)** is a water soluble prodrug of phenytoin. The advantages of fosphenytoin are faster loading and greater ease of administration. The dose of fosphenytoin is expressed in phenytoin equivalents (PE). The loading dose is 20 mg PE/kg IV at 150 mg/min, followed by 100 mg PE IV q8h. Fosphenytoin may be given IV or IM in normal saline or D5W.

C. Refractory status epilepticus

1. Intubation should be accomplished and blood pressure support should be maintained with fluids and pressor agents. EEG monitoring should be initiated.
2. **Midazolam (Versed)** should be administered if seizures continue. Loading dose is 0.2 mg/kg, followed by 0.045 mg/kg/hr. Titrate to 0.6 mg/kg/hr.
3. **Propofol (Diprivan)** may be used if midazolam (Versed) is ineffective. Loading dose is 1-2 mg/kg, followed by 2 mg/kg/hr, titrate to 10 mg/kg/hr. Adjust dose to achieve seizure-free status on EEG monitoring.
4. **Phenobarbital** may be administered as an alternative to anesthetics if the patient is not hypoxemic or hyperthermic and seizure activity is intermittent. The loading dose is 20 mg/kg at 75 mg/min, then 2 mg/kg IV q12h.

References

Brott T, et al. Treatment of Acute Ischemic Stroke. N Engl J Med 2000; 343:710-722.
Lowenstein DH, et al. Status epilepticus. N Engl J Med 1998; 338:970-976.

Endocrinologic and Nephrologic Disorders

Michael Krutzik, MD
Guy Foster, MD

Diabetic Ketoacidosis

Diabetic ketoacidosis is defined by hyperglycemia, metabolic acidosis, and ketosis.

I. **Clinical presentation**
   A. Diabetes is newly diagnosed in 20% of cases of diabetic ketoacidosis. In patients with known diabetes, precipitating factors include infection, noncompliance with insulin, myocardial infarction, and gastrointestinal bleeding.
   B. **Symptoms of DKA** include polyuria, polydipsia, fatigue, nausea, and vomiting, developing over 1 to 2 days. Abdominal pain is prominent in 25%.
   C. **Physical examination**
      1. Patients are typically flushed, tachycardic, tachypneic, and volume depleted with dry mucous membranes. Kussmaul's respiration (rapid, deep breathing and air hunger) occurs when the serum pH is between 7.0 and 7.24.
      2. **A fruity odor** on the breath indicates the presence of acetone, a byproduct of diabetic ketoacidosis.
      3. **Fever**, although seldom present, indicates infection. Eighty percent of patients with diabetic ketoacidosis have altered mental status. Most are awake but confused; 10% are comatose.
   D. **Laboratory findings**
      1. Serum glucose level >300 mg/dL
      2. pH <7.35, pCO_2 <40 mm Hg
      3. Bicarbonate level below normal with an elevated anion gap
      4. Presence of ketones in the serum
II. **Differential diagnosis**
   A. **Differential diagnosis of ketosis-causing conditions**
      1. **Alcoholic ketoacidosis** occurs with heavy drinking and vomiting. It does not cause an elevated glucose.
      2. **Starvation ketosis** occurs after 24 hours without food and is not usually confused with DKA because glucose and serum pH are normal.
   B. **Differential diagnosis of acidosis-causing conditions**
      1. **Metabolic acidoses** are divided into increased anion gap (>14 mEq/L) and normal anion gap; anion gap = sodium - ($Cl_- + HCO_3^-$).
      2. **Anion gap acidoses** can be caused by ketoacidoses, lactic acidosis, uremia, salicylate, methanol, ethanol, or ethylene glycol poisoning.
      3. **Non-anion gap acidoses** are associated with a normal glucose level and absent serum ketones. Causes of non-anion gap acidoses include renal or gastrointestinal bicarbonate loss.

C. **Hyperglycemia caused by hyperosmolar nonketotic coma** occurs in patients with type 2 diabetes with severe hyperglycemia. Patients are usually elderly and have a precipitating illness. Glucose level is markedly elevated (>600 mg/dL), osmolarity is increased, and ketosis is minimal.

III. Treatment of diabetic ketoacidosis

A. Fluid resuscitation

1. Fluid deficits average 5 liters or 50 mL/kg. Resuscitation consists of 1 liter of normal saline over the first hour and a second liter over the second and third hours. Thereafter, ½ normal saline should be infused at 100-120 mL/hr.

2. When the glucose level decreases to 250 mg/dL, 5% dextrose should be added to the replacement fluids to prevent hypoglycemia. If the glucose level declines rapidly, 10% dextrose should be infused along with regular insulin until the anion gap normalizes.

B. Insulin

1. An initial loading dose consists of 0.1 U/kg IV bolus. Insulin is then infused at 0.1 U/kg per hour. The biologic half-life of IV insulin is less than 20 minutes. The insulin infusion should be adjusted each hour so that the glucose decline does not exceed 100 mg/dL per hour.

2. The insulin infusion rate may be decreased when the bicarbonate level is greater than 20 mEq/L, the anion gap is less than 16 mEq/L, or the glucose is <250 mg/dL.

C. Potassium

1. The most common preventable cause of death in patients with DKA is hypokalemia. The typical deficit is between 300 and 500 mEq.

2. Potassium chloride should be started when fluid therapy is started. In most patients, the initial rate of potassium replacement is 20 mEq/h, but hypokalemia requires more aggressive replacement (40 mEq/h).

3. All patients should receive potassium replacement, except for those with renal failure, no urine output, or an initial serum potassium level greater than 6.0 mEq/L.

D. Sodium. For every 100 mg/dL that glucose is elevated, the sodium level should be assumed to be higher than the measured value by 1.6 mEq/L.

E. Phosphate. Diabetic ketoacidosis depletes phosphate stores. Serum phosphate level should be checked after 4 hours of treatment. If it is below 1.5 mg/dL, potassium phosphate should be added to the IV solution in place of KCl.

F. Bicarbonate therapy is not required unless the arterial pH value is <7.0. For a pH of <7.0, add 50 mEq of sodium bicarbonate to the first liter of IV fluid.

G. Magnesium. The usual magnesium deficit is 2-3 gm. If the patient's magnesium level is less than 1.8 mEq/L or if tetany is present, magnesium sulfate is given as 5g in 500 mL of 0.45% normal saline over 5 hours.

H. Additional therapies

1. A nasogastric tube should be inserted in semiconscious patients to protect against aspiration.

2. Deep vein thrombosis prophylaxis with subcutaneous heparin should be provided for patients who are elderly, unconscious, or severely hyperosmolar (5,000 U every 12 hours).

IV. Monitoring of therapy

A. Serum bicarbonate level and anion gap should be monitored to determine the effectiveness of insulin therapy.

B. **Glucose levels** should be checked at 1-2 hour intervals during IV insulin administration.

C. **Electrolyte levels** should be assessed every 2 hours for the first 6-8 hours, and then q8h. Phosphorus and magnesium levels should be checked after 4 hours of treatment.

D. **Plasma and urine ketones** are helpful in diagnosing diabetic ketoacidosis, but are not necessary during therapy.

V. **Determining the underlying cause**

A. **Infection** is the underlying cause of diabetic ketoacidosis in 50% of cases. Infection of the urinary tract, respiratory tract, skin, sinuses, ears, or teeth should be sought. Fever is unusual in diabetic ketoacidosis and indicates infection when present. If infection is suspected, antibiotics should be promptly initiated.

B. **Omission of insulin doses** is often a precipitating factor. Myocardial infarction, ischemic stroke, and abdominal catastrophes may precipitate DKA.

VI. **Initiation of subcutaneous insulin**

A. When the serum bicarbonate and anion gap levels are normal, subcutaneous regular insulin can be started.

B. Intravenous and subcutaneous administration of insulin should overlap to avoid redevelopment of ketoacidosis. The intravenous infusion may be stopped 1 hour after the first subcutaneous injection of insulin.

C. **Estimation of subcutaneous insulin requirements**

1. Multiply the final insulin infusion rate times 24 hours. Two-thirds of the total dose is given in the morning as two-thirds NPH and one-third regular insulin. The remaining one-third of the total dose is given before supper as one-half NPH and one-half regular insulin.

2. Subsequent doses should be adjusted according to the patient's blood glucose response.

Acute Renal Failure

Acute renal failure is defined as a sudden decrease in renal function sufficient to increase the concentration of nitrogenous wastes in the blood. It is characterized by an increasing BUN and creatinine.

I. **Clinical presentation of acute renal failure**

A. **Oliguria** is a common indicator of acute renal failure, and it is marked by a decrease in urine output to less than 30 mL/h. Acute renal failure may be oliguric (<500 L/day) or nonoliguric (>30 mL/h). Anuria (<100 mL/day) does not usually occur in renal failure, and its presence suggests obstruction or a vascular cause.

B. Acute renal failure may also be manifest by encephalopathy, volume overload, pericarditis, bleeding, anemia, hyperkalemia, hyperphosphatemia, hypocalcemia, and metabolic acidemia.

II. **Clinical causes of renal failure**

A. **Prerenal insult**

1. Prerenal insult is the most common cause of acute renal failure, accounting for 70% of cases. Prerenal failure is usually caused by reduced renal perfusion secondary to extracellular fluid loss (diarrhea, diuresis, GI hemorrhage) or secondary to extracellular fluid sequestra-

tion (pancreatitis, sepsis), inadequate cardiac output, renal vasoconstriction (sepsis, liver disease, drugs), or inadequate fluid intake or replacement.

2. Most patients with prerenal azotemia have oliguria, a history of large fluid losses (vomiting, diarrhea, burns), and evidence of intravascular volume depletion (thirst, weight loss, orthostatic hypotension, tachycardia, flat neck veins, dry mucous membranes). Patients with congestive heart failure may have total body volume excess (distended neck veins, pulmonary and pedal edema) but still have compromised renal perfusion and prerenal azotemia because of diminished cardiac output.

3. Causes of prerenal failure are usually reversible if recognized and treated early; otherwise, prolonged renal hypoperfusion can lead to acute tubular necrosis and permanent renal insufficiency.

B. **Intrarenal insult**

1. **Acute tubular necrosis (ATN)** is the most common intrinsic renal disease leading to ARF.

   a. **Prolonged renal hypoperfusion** is the most common cause of ATN.

   b. **Nephrotoxic agents** (aminoglycosides, heavy metals, radiocontrast media, ethylene glycol) represent exogenous nephrotoxins. ATN may also occur as a result of endogenous nephrotoxins, such as intratubular pigments (hemoglobinuria), intratubular proteins (myeloma), and intratubular crystals (uric acid).

2. **Acute interstitial nephritis (AIN)** is an allergic reaction secondary to drugs (NSAIDs, β-lactams).

3. **Arteriolar injury** occurs secondary to hypertension, vasculitis, microangiopathic disorders.

4. **Glomerulonephritis** secondary to immunologically mediated inflammation may cause intrarenal damage.

C. **Postrenal insult** results from obstruction of urine flow. Postrenal insult is the least common cause of acute renal failure, accounting for 10%. Postrenal insult may be caused by obstruction secondary to prostate cancer, benign prostatic hypertrophy, or renal calculi. Postrenal insult may be caused by amyloidosis, uric acid crystals, multiple myeloma, methotrexate, or acyclovir.

III. **Clinical evaluation of acute renal failure**

A. **Initial evaluation** of renal failure should determine whether the cause is decreased renal perfusion, obstructed urine flow, or disorders of the renal parenchyma. Volume status (orthostatic pulse, blood pressure, fluid intake and output, daily weights, hemodynamic parameters), nephrotoxic medications, and pattern of urine output should be assessed.

B. **Prerenal azotemia** is likely when there is a history of heart failure or extracellular fluid volume loss or depletion.

C. **Postrenal azotemia** is suggested by a history of decreased size or force of the urine stream, anuria, flank pain, hematuria or pyuria, or cancer of the bladder, prostate or pelvis.

D. **Intrarenal insult** is suggested by a history of prolonged volume depletion (often post-surgical), pigmenturia, hemolysis, rhabdomyolysis, or nephrotoxins. Intrarenal insult is suggested by recent radiocontrast, aminoglycoside use, or vascular catheterization. Interstitial nephritis may be implicated by a history of medication rash, fever, or arthralgias.

E. **Chronic renal failure** is suggested by diabetes mellitus, normochromic normocytic anemia, hypercalcemia, and hyperphosphatemia.

IV. **Physical examination**
   A. Cardiac output, volume status, bladder size, and systemic disease manifestations should be assessed.
   B. **Prerenal azotemia** is suggested by impaired cardiac output (neck vein distention, pulmonary rales, pedal edema). Volume depletion is suggested by orthostatic blood pressure changes, weight loss, low urine output, or diuretic use.
   C. **Flank, suprapubic, or abdominal masses** may indicate an obstructive cause.
   D. **Skin rash** suggests drug-induced interstitial nephritis; palpable purpura suggests vasculitis; nonpalpable purpura suggests thrombotic thrombocytopenic purpura or hemolytic-uremic syndrome.
   E. **Bladder catheterization** is useful to rule out suspected bladder outlet obstruction. A residual volume of more than 100 mL suggests bladder outlet obstruction.
   F. **Central venous monitoring** is used to measure cardiac output and left ventricular filling pressure if prerenal failure is suspected.

V. **Laboratory evaluation**
   A. **Spot urine sodium concentration**
      1. Spot urine sodium can help distinguish between prerenal azotemia and acute tubular necrosis.
      2. Prerenal failure causes increased reabsorption of salt and water and will manifest as a low spot urine sodium concentration <20 mEq/L and a low fractional sodium excretion <1%, and a urine/plasma creatinine ration of >40. Fractional excretion of sodium (%) = ([urine sodium/plasma sodium] ÷ [urine creatinine/plasma creatinine] x 100).
      3. If tubular necrosis is the cause, the spot urine concentration will be >40 mEq/L, and fractional excretion of sodium will be >1%.
   B. **Urinalysis**
      1. **Normal urine sediment** is a strong indicator of prerenal azotemia or may be an indicator of obstructive uropathy.
      2. **Hematuria, pyuria, or crystals** may be associated with postrenal obstructive azotemia.
      3. **Abundant cells, casts, or protein** suggests an intrarenal disorder.
      4. **Red cells** alone may indicate vascular disorders. RBC casts and abundant protein suggest glomerular disease (glomerulonephritis).
      5. **White cell casts and eosinophilic casts** indicate interstitial nephritis.
      6. **Renal epithelial cell casts and pigmented granular casts** are associated with acute tubular necrosis.
   C. **Ultrasound** is useful for evaluation of suspected postrenal obstruction (nephrolithiasis). The presence of small (<10 cm in length), scarred kidneys is diagnostic of chronic renal insufficiency.

VI. **Management of acute renal failure**
   A. Reversible disorders, such as obstruction, should be excluded, and hypovolemia should be corrected with volume replacement. Cardiac output should be maintained. In critically ill patients, a pulmonary artery catheter should be used for evaluation and monitoring.
   B. **Extracellular fluid volume expansion.** Infusion of a 1-2 liter crystalloid fluid bolus may confirm suspected volume depletion.
   C. If the patient remains oliguric despite euvolemia, IV diuretics may be administered. A large single dose of furosemide (100-200 mg) may be administered intravenously to promote diuresis. If urine flow is not improved, the dose of furosemide may be doubled. Furosemide may be

    repeated in 2 hours, or a continuous IV infusion of 10-40 mg/hr (max 1000 mg/day) may be used.

D. The dosage or dosing intervals of renally excreted drugs should be modified.

E. Hyperkalemia is the most immediately life-threatening complication of renal failure. Serum potassium values greater than 6.5 mEq/L may lead to arrhythmias and cardiac arrest. Potassium should be removed from IV solutions. Hyperkalemia may be treated with sodium polystyrene sulfonate (Kayexalate), 30-60 gm PO/PR every 4-6 hours.

F. Hyperphosphatemia can be controlled with aluminum hydroxide antacids (eg, Amphojel or Basaljel), 15-30 ml or one to three capsules PO with meals, should be used.

G. Fluids. After normal volume has been restored, fluid intake should be reduced to an amount equal to urinary and other losses plus insensible losses of 300-500 mL/day. In oliguric patients, daily fluid intake may need to be restricted to less than 1 L.

H. Nutritional therapy. A renal diet consisting of daily high biologic value protein intake of 0.5 gm/kg/d, sodium 2 g, potassium 40-60 mg/day, and at least 35 kcal/kg of nonprotein calories is recommended. Phosphorus should be restricted to 800 mg/day

I. Dialysis. Indications for dialysis include uremic pericarditis, severe hyperkalemia, pulmonary edema, persistent severe metabolic acidosis (pH less than 7.2), and symptomatic uremia.

Hyperkalemia

Body potassium is 98% intracellular. Only 2% of total body potassium, about 70 mEq, is in the extracellular fluid, with the normal concentration of 3.5-5 mEq/L.

I. Pathophysiology of potassium homeostasis
    A. The normal upper limit of plasma K is 5-5.5 mEq/L, with a mean K level of 4.3.
    B. External potassium balance. Normal dietary K intake is 1-1.5 mEq/kg in the form of vegetables and meats. The kidney is the primary organ for preserving external K balance, excreting 90% of the daily K burden.
    C. Internal potassium balance. Potassium transfer to and from tissues, is affected by insulin, acid-base status, catecholamines, aldosterone, plasma osmolality, cellular necrosis, and glucagon.

II. Clinical disorders of external potassium balance
    A. Chronic renal failure. The kidney is able to excrete the dietary intake of potassium until the glomerular filtration rate falls below 10 cc/minute or until urine output falls below 1 L/day. Renal failure is advanced before hyperkalemia occurs.
    B. Impaired renal tubular function. Renal diseases may cause hyperkalemia, and the renal tubular acidosis caused by these conditions may worsen hyperkalemia.
    C. Primary adrenal insufficiency (Addison's disease) is now a rare cause of hyperkalemia. Diagnosis is indicated by the combination of hyperkalemia and hyponatremia and is confirmed by a low aldosterone and a low plasma cortisol level that does not respond to adreno-corticotropic hormone treatment.

D. Drugs that may cause hyperkalemia include nonsteroidal anti-inflammatory drugs, angiotensin-converting enzyme inhibitors, cyclosporine, and potassium-sparing diuretics. Hyperkalemia is especially common when these drugs are given to patients at risk for hyperkalemia (diabetics, renal failure, advanced age).

E. Excessive potassium intake
   1. Long-term potassium supplementation results in hyperkalemia most often when an underlying impairment in renal excretion already exists.
   2. Intravenous administration of 0.5 mEq/kg over 1 hour increases serum levels by 0.6 mEq/L. Hyperkalemia often results when infusions of greater than 40 mEq/hour are given.

III. Clinical disorders of internal potassium balance
   A. Diabetic patients are at particular risk for severe hyperkalemia because of renal insufficiency and hyporeninemic hypoaldosteronism.
   B. Systemic acidosis reduces renal excretion of potassium and moves potassium out of cells, resulting in hyperkalemia.
   C. Endogenous potassium release from muscle injury, tumor lysis, or chemotherapy may elevate serum potassium.

IV. Manifestations of hyperkalemia
   A. Hyperkalemia, unless severe, is usually asymptomatic. The effect of hyperkalemia on the heart becomes significant above 6 mEq/L. As levels increase, the initial ECG change is tall peaked T waves. The QT interval is normal or diminished.
   B. As K levels rise further, the PR interval becomes prolonged, then the P wave amplitude decreases. The QRS complex eventually widens into a sine wave pattern, with subsequent cardiac standstill.
   C. At serum K is >7 mEq/L, muscle weakness may lead to a flaccid paralysis. Sensory abnormalities, impaired speech and respiratory arrest may follow.

V. Pseudohyperkalemia
   A. Potassium may be falsely elevated by hemolysis during phlebotomy, when K is released from ischemic muscle distal to a tourniquet, and because of erythrocyte fragility disorders.
   B. Falsely high laboratory measurement of serum potassium may occur with markedly elevated platelet counts ($>10^6$ platelet/mm^3) or white blood cell counts (>50,000/mm^3).

VI. Diagnostic approach to hyperkalemia
   A. The serum K level should be repeat tested to rule out laboratory error. If significant thrombocytosis or leukocytosis is present, a plasma potassium level should be determined.
   B. The 24-hour urine output, urinary K excretion, blood urea nitrogen, and serum creatinine should be measured. Renal K retention is diagnosed when urinary K excretion is less than 20 mEq/day.
   C. High urinary K, excretion of >20 mEq/day, is indicative of excessive K intake as the cause.

VII. Renal hyperkalemia
   A. If urinary K excretion is low and urine output is in the oliguric range, and creatinine clearance is lower than 20 cc/minute, renal failure is the probable cause. Prerenal azotemia resulting from volume depletion must be ruled out because the hyperkalemia will respond to volume restoration.
   B. When urinary K excretion is low, yet blood urea nitrogen and creatinine levels are not elevated and urine volume is at least 1 L daily and renal

sodium excretion is adequate (about 20 mEq/day), then either a defect in the secretion of renin or aldosterone or tubular resistance to aldosterone is likely. Low plasma renin and aldosterone levels, will confirm the diagnosis of hyporeninemic hypoaldosteronism. Addison's disease is suggested by a low serum cortisol, and the diagnosis is confirmed with a ACTH (Cortrosyn) stimulation test.

C. When inadequate K excretion is not caused by hypoaldosteronism, a tubular defect in K clearance is suggested. Urinary tract obstruction, renal transplant, lupus, or a medication should be considered.

VIII. **Extrarenal hyperkalemia**

A. When hyperkalemia occurs along with high urinary K excretion of >20 mEq/day, excessive intake of K is the cause. Potassium excess in IV fluids, diet, or medication should be sought. A concomitant underlying renal defect in K excretion is also likely to be present.

B. Blood sugar should be measured to rule out insulin deficiency; blood pH and serum bicarbonate should be measured to rule out acidosis.

C. Endogenous sources of K, such as tissue necrosis, hypercatabolism, hematoma, gastrointestinal bleeding, or intravascular hemolysis should be excluded.

IX. **Management of hyperkalemia**

A. **Acute treatment of hyperkalemia**

1. **Calcium**

   a. If the electrocardiogram shows loss of P waves or widening of QRS complexes, calcium should be given IV; calcium reduces the cell membrane threshold potential.

   b. Calcium chloride (10%) 2-3 g should be given over 5 minutes. In patients with circulatory compromise, 1 g of calcium chloride IV should be given over 3 minutes.

   c. If the serum K level is greater than 7 mEq/L, calcium should be given. If digitalis intoxication is suspected, calcium must be given cautiously. Coexisting hyponatremia should be treated with hypertonic saline.

2. **Insulin:** If the only ECG abnormalities are peaked T waves and the serum level is under 7 mEq/L, treatment should begin with insulin (regular insulin, 5-10 U by IV push) with 50% dextrose water (D50W) 50 mL IV push. Repeated insulin doses of 10 U and glucose can be given every 15 minutes for maximal effect.

3. **Sodium bicarbonate** promotes cellular uptake of K. It should be given as 1-2 vials (50-mEq/vials) IV push.

4. **Potassium elimination measures**

   a. Sodium polystyrene sulfonate (Kayexalate) is a cation exchange resin which binds to potassium in the lower GI tract. Dosage is 30-60 gm premixed with sorbitol 20% PO/PR.

   b. Furosemide (Lasix) 100 mg IV should be given to promote kaliuresis.

   c. Emergent hemodialysis for hyperkalemia is rarely necessary except when refractory metabolic acidosis is present.

Hypokalemia

Hypokalemia is characterized by a serum potassium concentration of less than 3.5 mEq/L. Ninety-eight percent of K is intracellular.

I. Pathophysiology of hypokalemia
  A. **Cellular redistribution of potassium.** Hypokalemia may result from the intracellular shift of potassium by insulin, beta-2 agonist drugs, stress induced catecholamine release, thyrotoxic periodic paralysis, and alkalosis-induced shift (metabolic or respiratory).
  B. **Nonrenal potassium loss**
    1. Gastrointestinal loss can be caused by diarrhea, laxative abuse, villous adenoma, biliary drainage, enteric fistula, clay ingestion, potassium binding resin ingestion, or nasogastric suction.
    2. Sweating, prolonged low-potassium diet, hemodialysis and peritoneal dialysis may also cause nonrenal potassium loss.
  C. **Renal potassium loss**
    1. **Hypertensive high renin states.** Malignant hypertension, renal artery stenosis, renin-producing tumors.
    2. **Hypertensive low renin, high aldosterone states.** Primary hyperaldosteronism (adenoma or hyperplasia).
    3. **Hypertensive low renin, low aldosterone states.** Congenital adrenal hyperplasia (11 or 17 hydroxylase deficiency), Cushing's syndrome or disease, exogenous mineralocorticoids (Florinef, licorice, chewing tobacco), Liddle's syndrome.
    4. **Normotensive states**
      a. **Metabolic acidosis.** Renal tubular acidosis (type I or II)
      b. **Metabolic alkalosis (urine chloride <10 mEq/day).** Vomiting
      c. **Metabolic alkalosis (urine chloride >10 mEq/day).** Bartter's syndrome, diuretics, magnesium depletion, normotensive hyper-aldosteronism
    5. **Drugs** associated with potassium loss include amphotericin B, ticarcillin, piperacillin, and loop diuretics.
II. Clinical effects of hypokalemia
  A. **Cardiac effects.** The most lethal consequence of hypokalemia is cardiac arrhythmia. Electrocardiographic effects include a depressed ST segment, decreased T-wave amplitude, U waves, and a prolonged QT-U interval.
  B. **Musculoskeletal effects.** The initial manifestation of K depletion is muscle weakness, which can lead to paralysis. In severe cases, respiratory muscle paralysis may occur.
  C. **Gastrointestinal effects.** Nausea, vomiting, constipation, and paralytic ileus may develop.
III. Diagnostic evaluation
  A. The 24-hour urinary potassium excretion should be measured. If >20 mEq/day, excessive urinary K loss is the cause. If <20 mEq/d, low K intake, or non-urinary K loss is the cause.
  B. In patients with excessive renal K loss and hypertension, plasma renin and aldosterone should be measured to differentiate adrenal from non-adrenal causes of hyperaldosteronism.
  C. If hypertension is absent and serum pH is acidotic, renal tubular acidosis should be considered. If hypertension is absent and serum pH is normal

to alkalotic, a high urine chloride (>10 mEq/d) suggests hypokalemia secondary to diuretics or Bartter's syndrome. A low urine chloride (<10 mEq/d) suggests vomiting.

IV. **Emergency treatment of hypokalemia**
   A. **Indications for urgent replacement.** Electrocardiographic abnormalities, myocardial infarction, hypoxia, digitalis intoxication, marked muscle weakness, or respiratory muscle paralysis.
   B. **Intravenous potassium therapy**
      1. Intravenous KCL is usually used unless concomitant hypophosphatemia is present, where potassium phosphate is indicated.
      2. The maximal rate of intravenous K replacement is 30 mEq/hour. The K concentration of IV fluids should be 80 mEq/L or less if given via a peripheral vein. Frequent monitoring of serum K and constant electrocardiographic monitoring is recommended when potassium levels are being replaced.

V. **Non-emergent treatment of hypokalemia**
   A. Attempts should be made to normalize K levels if <3.5 mEq/L.
   B. Oral supplementation is significantly safer than IV. Liquid formulations are preferred due to rapid oral absorption, compared to sustained release formulations, which are absorbed over several hours.
      1. KCL elixir 20-40 mEq qd-tid PO after meals.
      2. Micro-K, 10 mEq tabs, 2-3 tabs tid PO after meals (40-100 mEq/d).

Hypomagnesemia

Magnesium deficiency occurs in up to 11% of hospitalized patients. The normal range of serum magnesium is 1.5 to 2.0 mEq/L, which is maintained by the kidney, intestine, and bone.

I. **Pathophysiology**
   A. **Decreased magnesium intake.** Protein-calorie malnutrition, prolonged parenteral fluid administration, and catabolic illness are common causes of hypomagnesemia.
   B. **Gastrointestinal losses of magnesium** may result from prolonged nasogastric suction, laxative abuse, and pancreatitis.
   C. **Renal losses of magnesium**
      1. Renal loss of magnesium may occur secondary to renal tubular acidosis, glomerulonephritis, interstitial nephritis, or acute tubular necrosis.
      2. Hyperthyroidism, hypercalcemia, and hypophosphatemia may cause magnesium loss.
      3. **Agents that enhance renal magnesium excretion** include alcohol, loop and thiazide diuretics, amphotericin B, aminoglycosides, cisplatin, and pentamidine.
   D. **Alterations in magnesium distribution**
      1. Redistribution of circulating magnesium occurs by extracellular to intracellular shifts, sequestration, hungry bone syndrome, or by acute administration of glucose, insulin, or amino acids.
      2. Magnesium depletion can be caused by large quantities of parenteral fluids and pancreatitis-induced sequestration of magnesium.

II. Clinical manifestations of hypomagnesemia

A. **Neuromuscular findings** may include positive Chvostek's and Trousseau's signs, tremors, myoclonic jerks, seizures, and coma.

B. **Cardiovascular.** Ventricular tachycardia, ventricular fibrillation, atrial fibrillation, multifocal atrial tachycardia, ventricular ectopic beats, hypertension, enhancement of digoxin-induced dysrhythmias, and cardiomyopathies.

C. **ECG changes** include ventricular arrhythmias (extrasystoles, tachycardia) and atrial arrhythmias (atrial fibrillation, supraventricular tachycardia, torsades de Pointes). Prolonged PR and QT intervals, ST segment depression, T-wave inversions, wide QRS complexes, and tall T-waves may occur.

III. Clinical evaluation

A. Hypomagnesemia is diagnosed when the serum magnesium is less than 0.7-0.8 mmol/L. Symptoms of magnesium deficiency occur when the serum magnesium concentration is less than 0.5 mmol/L. A 24-hour urine collection for magnesium is the first step in the evaluation of hypomagnesemia. Hypomagnesia caused by renal magnesium loss is associated with magnesium excretion that exceeds 24 mg/day.

B. Low urinary magnesium excretion (<1 mmol/day), with concomitant serum hypomagnesemia, suggests magnesium deficiency due to decreased intake, nonrenal losses, or redistribution of magnesium.

IV. Treatment of hypomagnesemia

A. **Asymptomatic magnesium deficiency**

1. In hospitalized patients, the daily magnesium requirements can be provided through either a balanced diet, as oral magnesium supplements (0.36-0.46 mEq/kg/day), or 16-30 mEq/day in a parenteral nutrition formulation.

2. Magnesium oxide is better absorbed and less likely to cause diarrhea than magnesium sulfate. Magnesium oxide preparations include Mag-Ox 400 (240 mg elemental magnesium per 400 mg tablet), Uro-Mag (84 mg elemental magnesium per 400 mg tablet), and magnesium chloride (Slo-Mag) 64 mg/tab, 1-2 tabs bid.

B. **Symptomatic magnesium deficiency**

1. Serum magnesium ≤0.5 mmol/L requires IV magnesium repletion with electrocardiographic and respiratory monitoring.

2. Magnesium sulfate 1-6 gm in 500 mL of D5W can be infused IV at 1 gm/hr. An additional 6-9 gm of $MgSO_4$ should be given by continuous infusion over the next 24 hours.

Hypermagnesemia

Serum magnesium has a normal range of 0.8-1.2 mmol/L. Magnesium homeostasis is regulated by renal and gastrointestinal mechanisms. Hypermagnesemia is usually iatrogenic and is frequently seen in conjunction with renal insufficiency.

I. Clinical evaluation of hypermagnesemia

A. **Causes of hypermagnesemia**

1. **Renal.** Creatinine clearance <30 mL/minute.

2. **Nonrenal.** Excessive use of magnesium cathartics, especially with renal failure; iatrogenic overtreatment with magnesium sulfate.

B. **Cardiovascular manifestations of hypermagnesemia**
   1. **Hypermagnesemia <10 mEq/L.** Delayed interventricular conduction, first-degree heart block, prolongation of the Q-T interval.
   2. **Levels greater than 10 mEq/L.** Low-grade heart block progressing to complete heart block and asystole occurs at levels greater than 12.5 mmol/L (>6.25 mmol/L).

C. **Neuromuscular effects**
   1. Hyporeflexia occurs at a magnesium level >4 mEq/L (>2 mmol/L); diminution of deep tendon reflexes is an early sign of magnesium toxicity.
   2. Respiratory depression due to respiratory muscle paralysis, somnolence and coma occur at levels >13 mEq/L (6.5 mmol/L).
   3. Hypermagnesemia should always be considered when these symptoms occur in patients with renal failure, in those receiving therapeutic magnesium, and in laxative abuse.

II. **Treatment of hypermagnesemia**
A. **Asymptomatic, hemodynamically stable patients.** Moderate hypermagnesemia can be managed by elimination of intake.

B. **Severe hypermagnesemia**
   1. Furosemide 20-40 mg IV q3-4h should be given as needed. Saline diuresis should be initiated with 0.9% saline, infused at 120 cc/h to replace urine loss.
   2. If ECG abnormalities (peaked T waves, loss of P waves, or widened QRS complexes) or if respiratory depression is present, IV calcium gluconate should be given as 1-3 ampules (10% solution, 1 gm per 10 mL amp), added to saline infusate. Calcium gluconate can be infused to reverse acute cardiovascular toxicity or respiratory failure as 15 mg/kg over a 4-hour period.
   3. Parenteral insulin and glucose can be given to shift magnesium into cells. Dialysis is necessary for patients who have severe hypermagnesemia.

Disorders of Water and Sodium Balance

I. **Pathophysiology of water and sodium balance**
A. Volitional intake of water is regulated by thirst. Maintenance intake of water is the amount of water sufficient to offset obligatory losses.

B. **Maintenance water needs**
   = 100 mL/kg for first 10 kg of body weight
   + 50 mL/kg for next 10 kg
   + 20 mL/kg for weight greater than 20 kg

C. **Clinical signs of hyponatremia.** Confusion, agitation, lethargy, seizures, and coma.

D. **Pseudohyponatremia**
   1. Elevation of blood glucose may creates an osmotic gradient that pulls water from cells into the extracellular fluid, diluting the extracellular sodium. The contribution of hyperglycemia to hyponatremia can be estimated using the following formula:
   Expected change in serum sodium = (serum glucose - 100) x 0.016

2. Marked elevation of plasma lipids or protein can also result in erroneous hyponatremia because of laboratory inaccuracy. The percentage of plasma water can be estimated with the following formula:

% plasma water = 100 - [0.01 x lipids (mg/dL)] - [0.73 x protein (g/dL)]

II. Diagnostic evaluation of hyponatremia

A. Pseudohyponatremia should be excluded by repeat testing. The cause of the hyponatremia should be determined based on history, physical exam, urine osmolality, serum osmolality, urine sodium and chloride. An assessment of volume status should determine if the patient is volume contracted, normal volume, or volume expanded.

B. Classification of hyponatremic patients based on urine osmolality

1. **Low-urine osmolality (50-180 mOsm/L)** indicates primary excessive water intake (psychogenic water drinking).

2. **High-urine osmolality (urine osmolality >serum osmolality)**

   a. **High-urine sodium (>40 mEq/L) and volume contraction** indicates a renal source of sodium loss and fluid loss (excessive diuretic use, salt-wasting nephropathy, Addison's disease, osmotic diuresis).

   b. **High-urine sodium (>40 mEq/L) and normal volume** is most likely caused by water retention due to a drug effect, hypothyroidism, or the syndrome of inappropriate antidiuretic hormone secretion. In SIADH, the urine sodium level is usually high. SIADH is found in the presence of a malignant tumor or a disorder of the pulmonary or central nervous system.

   c. **Low-urine sodium (<20 mEq/L) and volume contraction,** dry mucous membranes, decreased skin turgor, and orthostatic hypotension indicate an extrarenal source of fluid loss (gastrointestinal disease, burns).

   d. **Low-urine sodium (<20 mEq/L) and volume-expansion, and edema** is caused by congestive heart failure, cirrhosis with ascites, or nephrotic syndrome. Effective arterial blood volume is decreased. Decreased renal perfusion causes increased reabsorption of water.

Drugs Associated with SIADH

Acetaminophen	Isoproterenol
Barbiturates	Prostaglandin E$_1$
Carbamazepine	Meperidine
Chlorpropamide	Nicotine
Clofibrate	Tolbutamide
Cyclophosphamide	Vincristine
Indomethacin	

III. Treatment of water excess hyponatremia

A. Determine the volume of water excess

Water excess = total body water x ([140/measured sodium] -1)

B. Treatment of asymptomatic hyponatremia. Water intake should be restricted to 1,000 mL/day. Food alone in the diet contains this much water, so no liquids should be consumed. If an intravenous solution is needed, an isotonic solution of 0.9% sodium chloride (normal saline) should be used. Dextrose should not be used in the infusion because the dextrose is metabolized into water.

C. Treatment of symptomatic hyponatremia

1. If neurologic symptoms of hyponatremia are present, the serum sodium level should be corrected with hypertonic saline. Excessively rapid correction of sodium may result in a syndrome of central pontine demyelination.

2. The serum sodium should be raised at a rate of 1 mEq/L per hour. If hyponatremia has been chronic, the rate should be limited to 0.5 mEq/L per hour. The goal of initial therapy is a serum sodium of 125-130 mEq/L, then water restriction should be continued until the level normalizes.

3. The amount of hypertonic saline needed is estimated using the following formula:
   Sodium needed (mEq) = 0.6 x wt in kg x (desired sodium - measured sodium)

4. Hypertonic 3% sodium chloride contains 513 mEq/L of sodium. The calculated volume required should be administered over the period required to raise the serum sodium level at a rate of 0.5-1 mEq/L per hour. Concomitant administration of furosemide may be required to lessen the risk of fluid overload.

IV. Hypernatremia

A. Clinical manifestations of hypernatremia:
Clinical manifestations include tremulousness, irritability, ataxia, spasticity, mental confusion, seizures, and coma.

B. Causes of hypernatremia

1. Net sodium gain or net water loss will cause hypernatremia

2. Failure to replace obligate water losses may cause hypernatremia, as in patients unable to obtain water because of an altered mental status or severe debilitating disease.

3. **Diabetes insipidus:** If urine volume is high but urine osmolality is low, diabetes insipidus is the most likely cause.

Drugs Associated with Diabetes Insipidus	
Ethanol	Tolazamide
Phenytoin	Glyburide
Chlorpromazine	Amphotericin B
Lithium	Colchicine
Demeclocycline	Vinblastine

C. Diagnosis of hypernatremia

1. Assessment of urine volume and osmolality are essential in the evaluation of hyperosmolality. The usual renal response to hypernatremia is the excretion of the minimum volume (≤500 mL/day) of maximally concentrated urine (urine osmolality >800 mOsm/kg). These findings suggest extrarenal water loss.

2. Diabetes insipidus generally presents with polyuria and hypotonic urine (urine osmolality <250 mOsm/kg).

V. Management of hypernatremia

A. If there is evidence of hemodynamic compromise (eg, orthostatic hypotension, marked oliguria), fluid deficits should be corrected initially

with isotonic saline. Once hemodynamic stability is achieved, the remaining free water deficit should be corrected with 5% dextrose water or 0.45% NaCl.

B. The water deficit can be estimated using the following formula:

Water deficit = 0.6 x wt in kg x (1 - [140/measured sodium]).

C. The change in sodium concentration should not exceed 1 mEq/liter/hour. One-half of the calculated water deficit can be administered in the first 24 hours, followed by correction of the remaining deficit over the next 1-2 days. The serum sodium concentration and ECF volume status should be evaluated every 6 hours. Excessively rapid correction of hypernatremia may lead to lethargy and seizures secondary to cerebral edema.

D. Maintenance fluid needs from ongoing renal and insensible losses must also be provided. If the patient is conscious and able to drink, water should be given orally or by nasogastric tube.

E. Treatment of diabetes insipidus

1. **Vasopressin (Pitressin)** 5-10 U IV/SQ q6h; fast onset of action with short duration.
2. **Desmopressin (DDAVP)** 2-4 mcg IV/SQ q12h; slow onset of action with long duration of effect.

VI. Mixed disorders

A. Water excess and saline deficit occurs when severe vomiting and diarrhea occur in a patient who is given only water. Clinical signs of volume contraction and a low serum sodium are present. Saline deficit is replaced and free water intake restricted until the serum sodium level has normalized.

B. Water and saline excess often occurs with heart failure, manifesting as edema and a low serum sodium. An increase in the extracellular fluid volume, as evidenced by edema, is a saline excess. A marked excess of free water expands the extracellular fluid volume, causing apparent hyponatremia. However, the important derangement in edema is an excess of sodium. Sodium and water restriction and use of furosemide are usually indicated in addition to treatment of the underlying disorder.

C. Water and saline deficit is frequently caused by vomiting and high fever and is characterized by signs of volume contraction and an elevated serum sodium. Saline and free water should be replaced in addition to maintenance amounts of water.

Hypercalcemic Crisis

Hypercalcemic crisis is defined as an elevation in serum calcium that is associated with volume depletion, mental status changes, and life-threatening cardiac arrhythmias. Hypercalcemic crisis is most commonly caused by malignancy-associated bone resorption.

I. Diagnosis

A. Hypercalcemic crisis is often complicated by nausea, vomiting, hypovolemia, mental status changes, and hypotension.

B. A correction for the low albumin level must be made because ionized calcium is the physiologically important form of calcium.

Corrected serum calcium (mg/dL) = serum calcium + 0.8 x (4.0 - albumin [g/dL])

C. Most patients in hypercalcemic crisis have a corrected serum calcium level greater than 13 mg/dL.
D. The ECG often demonstrates a short QT interval. Bradyarrhythmias, heart blocks, and cardiac arrest may also occur.

II. **Treatment of hypercalcemic crisis**
A. Normal saline should be administered until the patient is normovolemic. If signs of fluid overload develop, furosemide (Lasix) can be given to promote sodium and calcium diuresis. Thiazide diuretics, vitamin D supplements and antacids containing sodium bicarbonate should be discontinued.
B. Pamidronate disodium (Aredia) is the agent of choice for long-term treatment of hypercalcemia. A single dose of 90-mg infused IV over 24 hours should normalize calcium levels in 4 to 7 days. The pamidronate dose of 30- to 90-mg IV infusion may be repeated 7 days after the initial dose. Smaller doses (30 or 60 mg IV over 4 hours) are given every few weeks to maintain normal calcium levels.
C. Calcitonin (Calcimar, Miacalcin) has the advantage of decreasing serum calcium levels within hours; 4 to 8 U/kg SQ/IM q12h. Calcitonin should be used in conjunction with pamidronate in severely hypercalcemic patients.

Hypophosphatemia

Clinical manifestations of hypophosphatemia include heart failure, muscle weakness, tremor, ataxia, seizures, coma, respiratory failure, delayed weaning from ventilator, hemolysis, and rhabdomyolysis.

I. **Differential diagnosis of hypophosphatemia**
A. Increased urinary excretion: Hyperparathyroidism, renal tubular defects, diuretics.
B. Decrease in GI absorption: Malnutrition, malabsorption, phosphate binding minerals (aluminum-containing antacids).
C. Abnormal vitamin D metabolism: Vitamin D deficiency, familial hypophosphatemia, tumor-associated hypercalcemia.
D. Intracellular shifts of phosphate: Diabetic ketoacidosis, respiratory alkalosis, alcohol withdrawal, recovery phase of starvation.

II. **Labs:** Phosphate, SMA 12, LDH, magnesium, calcium, albumin, PTH, urine electrolytes. 24-hr urine phosphate, and creatinine.

III. **Diagnostic approach to hypophosphatemia**
A. **24-hr urine phosphate**
1. If 24-hour urine phosphate is less than 100 mg/day, the cause is gastrointestinal losses (emesis, diarrhea, NG suction, phosphate binders), vitamin D deficit, refeeding, recovery from burns, alkalosis, alcoholism, or DKA.
2. If 24-hour urine phosphate is greater than 100 mg/day, the cause is renal losses, hyperparathyroidism, hypomagnesemia, hypokalemia, acidosis, diuresis, renal tubular defects, or vitamin D deficiency.

IV. Treatment

A. Mild hypophosphatemia (1.0-2.5 mEq/dL)

1. Na or K phosphate 0.25 mMol/kg IV infusion at the rate of 10 mMol/hr (in NS or D5W 150-250 mL), may repeat as needed.
2. Neutral phosphate (Nutra-Phos), 2 packs PO bid-tid (250 mg elemental phosphorus/pack).

B. Severe hypophosphatemia (<1.0 mEq/dL)

1. Administer Na or K phosphate 0.5 m Moles/Kg IV infusion at the rate of 10 mMoles/hr (NS or D5W 150-250 mL), may repeat as needed.
2. Add potassium phosphate to IV solution in place of KCl (max 80 mEq/L infused at 100-150 mL/h). Max IV dose 7.5 mg phosphorus/kg/6h OR 2.5-5 mg elemental phosphorus/kg IV over 6h. Give as potassium or sodium phosphate (93 mg phosphate/mL and 4 mEq Na+ or K+/mL). Do not mix calcium and phosphorus in same IV.

Hyperphosphatemia

I. Clinical manifestations of hyperphosphatemia: Hypotension, bradycardia, arrhythmias, bronchospasm, apnea, laryngeal spasm, tetany, seizures, weakness, psychosis, confusion.

II. Clinical evaluation of hyperphosphatemia

A. Exogenous phosphate administration: Enemas, laxatives, diphosphonates, vitamin D excess.

B. Endocrine disturbances: Hypoparathyroidism, acromegaly, PTH resistance.

C. Labs: Phosphate, SMA 12, calcium, parathyroid hormone. 24-hr urine phosphate, creatinine.

III. Therapy: Correct hypocalcemia, restrict dietary phosphate, saline diuresis.

A. Moderate hyperphosphatemia

1. Aluminum hydroxide (Amphojel) 5-10 mL or 1-2 tablets PO ac tid; aluminum containing agents bind to intestinal phosphate, and decreases absorption OR
2. Aluminum carbonate (Basaljel) 5-10 mL or 1-2 tablets PO ac tid OR
3. Calcium carbonate (Oscal) (250 or 500 mg elemental calcium/tab) 1-2 gm elemental calcium PO ac tid. Keep calcium-phosphate product <70; start only if phosphate <5.5.

B. Severe hyperphosphatemia

1. Volume expansion with 0.9% saline 1 L over 1h if the patient is not azotemic.
2. Dialysis is recommended for patients with renal failure.

References

Al-Shamadi SM, Cameron EC, Sutton RA, AW. J. Kidney Dis 1994; 24:737-52

De Marchi S, Cecchin E, Banile A, Bertotti A: NEJM 1993; 329: 1927-34

Berger W, Keller U: Treatment of diabetic ketoacidosis and non-ketotic hyperosmolar diabetic coma. Baillieres Clin Endo and Metab, Jan, 6(1):1, 1992.

Commonly Used Formulas

A-a gradient = $[(P_B - PH_2O) FiO_2 - PCO_2/R] - PO_2$ arterial

$$= (713 \times FiO_2 - pCO_2/0.8) - pO_2 \text{ arterial}$$

P_B = 760 mm Hg; PH_2O = 47 mm Hg; $R \approx 0.8$
normal Aa gradient <10-15 mm Hg (room air)

Arterial O_2 content = $1.36(Hgb)(SaO_2) + 0.003(PaO_2)$

O_2 delivery = CO x arterial O_2 content

Cardiac output = HR x stroke volume
Normal CO = 4-6 L/min

SVR = $\dfrac{MAP-CVP}{CO_{L/min}}$ x 80 = NL 800-1200 dyne/sec/cm^2

PVR = $\dfrac{PA-PCWP}{CO_{L/min}}$ x 80 = NL 45-120 dyne/sec/cm^2

Normal creatinine clearance = 100-125 mL/min(males), 85-105(females)

Body water deficit (L) = $\dfrac{0.6(\text{weight kg})([\text{measured serum Na}]-140)}{140}$

Osmolality mOsm/kg = $2[Na+ K] + \dfrac{BUN}{2.8} + \dfrac{glucose}{18}$ = NL 270-290 $\dfrac{mOsm}{kg}$

Fractional excreted Na = $\dfrac{U\ Na/\ Serum\ Na \times 100}{U\ Cr/\ Serum\ Cr}$ = NL<1%

Anion Gap = $Na + K - (Cl + HCO_3)$

For each 100 mg/dL ↑ in glucose, Na+ ↓ by 1.6 mEq/L.

Corrected serum Ca$^+$ (mg/dL) = measured Ca mg/dL + 0.8 x (4-albumin g/dL)

Basal energy expenditure (BEE):
  Males=66 + (13.7 x actual weight Kg) + (5 x height cm)-(6.8 x age)
  Females= 655+(9.6 x actual weight Kg)+(1.7 x height cm)-(4.7 x age)

Nitrogen Balance = Gm protein intake/6.25-urine urea nitrogen-(3-4 gm/d insensible loss)

Commonly Used Drug Levels

Drug	Therapeutic Range*
Amikacin	Peak 25-30; trough <10 mcg/mL
Amiodarone	1.0-3.0 mcg/mL
Amitriptyline	100-250 ng/mL
Carbamazepine	4-10 mcg/mL
Chloramphenicol	Peak 10-15; trough <5 mcg/mL
Desipramine	150-300 ng/mL
Digoxin	0.8-2.0 ng/mL
Disopyramide	2-5 mcg/mL
Doxepin	75-200 ng/mL
Flecainide	0.2-1.0 mcg/mL
Gentamicin	Peak 6.0-8.0; trough <2.0 mcg/mL

```
Imipramine ............ 150-300 ng/mL
Lidocaine ............. 2-5 mcg/mL
Lithium ............... 0.5-1.4 mEq/L
Nortriptyline ......... 50-150 ng/mL
Phenobarbital ......... 10-30 mEq/mL
Phenytoin** ........... 8-20 mcg/mL
Procainamide .......... 4.0-8.0 mcg/mL
Quinidine ............. 2.5-5.0 mcg/mL
Salicylate ............ 15-25 mg/dL
Theophylline .......... 8-20 mcg/mL
Valproic acid ......... 50-100 mcg/mL
Vancomycin ........... Peak 30-40; trough <10 mcg/mL
```

* The therapeutic range of some drugs may vary depending on the reference lab used.
** Therapeutic range of phenytoin is 4-10 mcg/mL in presence of significant azotemia and/or hypoalbuminemia.

Index